A COMPLETE GUIDE TO
MASSAGE

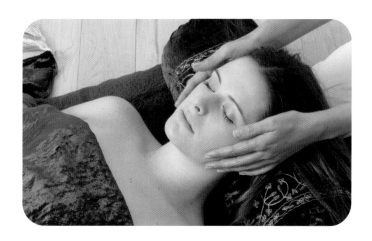

A COMPLETE GUIDE TO
MASSAGE

DENISE WHICHELLO BROWN

FOR GARRY, CHLÓE AND TOM

Published by SILVERDALE BOOKS
An imprint of Bookmart Ltd
Registered number 2372865
Trading as Bookmart Ltd
Desford Road
Enderby
Leicester LE19 4AD

© 2003 D&S Books Ltd

D&S Books Ltd
Kerswell,
Parkham Ash, Bideford
Devon, England
EX39 5PR

e-mail us at:-
enquiries@dsbooks.fsnet.co.uk

This edition printed 2003

ISBN 1-856057-39-9

Book code DS0067 Massage

Fonts used in this book: Helvetica

Creative Director: Sarah King
Editor: Judith Millidge
Project editor: Anna Southgate
Photographer: Colin Bowling
Designer: Axis Design Editions

Printed in China

1 3 5 7 9 10 8 6 4 2

CONTENTS

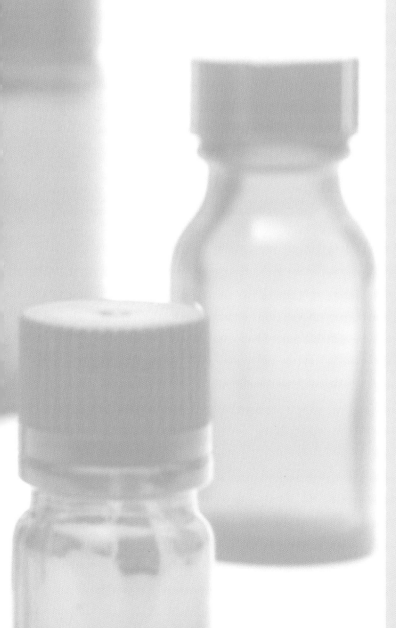

INTRODUCTION

THE IMPORTANCE OF TOUCH

MASSAGE FULFILS A BASIC HUMAN NEED –
IT SATISFIES THE DESIRE THAT WE ALL
HAVE BOTH TO TOUCH AND TO
BE TOUCHED.

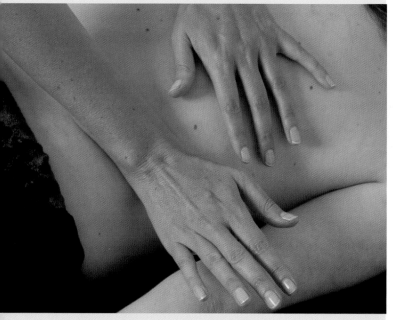

Touch is a fundamental human instinct, yet in the West social inhibitions mean that we touch each other very little. We tend to turn our attention to our pets and children. Indeed, we spend hours stroking our pets and research indicates that this relaxes us, reduces blood pressure and encourages the release of endorphins ('happy hormones') inducing a sense of well-being. It is also acceptable for parents to stroke and hug their children. This is pleasurable and comforting not only for the child, but for the adult too.

A parent will automatically rub a child's abdomen to soothe a tummy ache, rub a sore knee and soothe a fevered brow. In the majority of families, however, as children grow up, touch diminishes particularly around the onset of puberty when physical contact is often reduced to a bare minimum. Adolescents become embarrassed at this time when their bodies are developing and sexual desires are awakening; they may associate touch with sex rather then with love and healing. Thankfully, after this difficult and confusing stage of their development they usually come round to the idea that touching is acceptable! Through the language of touch we are able to express ourselves in a way that we never can through the spoken word. To hold someone's hand or to put an arm around a friend's shoulder is to let them know that we care and are there to support them. This reassurance is enormously important. It makes us feel valued, and transforms us both physically and psychologically.

THE HISTORY AND DEVELOPMENT OF MASSAGE

MASSAGE IS UNDOUBTEDLY THE OLDEST FORM OF PHYSICAL MEDICINE KNOWN TO MAN. IT HAS BEEN EMPLOYED FOR CENTURIES AS A NATURAL AND INSTINCTIVE WAY OF RELIEVING PAIN AND DISCOMFORT.

No one is exactly sure where and when the word massage originated, but there are several theories. In Greek *massein/masso* means to touch, handle, knead or squeeze. The Arabic, *mass/mass'h* means to press softly. The Latin *massa* means to touch, handle, knead or squeeze. In Sanskrit *makeh* means to press softly, and the French verb *masser* means to rub.

ANCIENT GREECE

Massage was widely practised in ancient Greece. In the 5th century BC Hippocrates, the Greek physician known as the 'father of medicine', strongly advocated the use of massage, noting that 'The physician must be acquainted with many things and assuredly with rubbing, for things which have the same name have not always the same effects, for rubbing can bind a joint that is too loose and loosen a joint that is too rigid... hard rubbing binds, much rubbing causes parts to waste and moderate rubbing makes them grow'.

The Greek physician Asclepiades who lived in the 1st century BC, used massage to treat his patients in conjunction with relaxation, diet, exercise and bathing. He taught that disease occurs due to an imbalance in the natural harmony of the body.

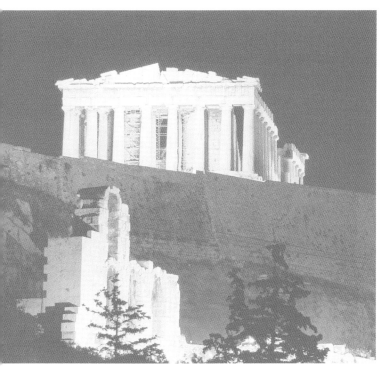

THE ANCIENT GREEKS WERE STRONG ADVOCATES OF THE USE OF MASSAGE.

ANCIENT ROME

Roman physicians used massage as a primary method of healing and relieving pain.

The Roman emperors' physician, Galen, (*c.* AD 130–201) prescribed massage for injured gladiators and also as preparation for combat. A firm believer in the use of massage, he wrote: 'Massage eliminates the waste products of nutrition and the poisons of fatigue.'

The Roman physician and writer Aulus Cornelius Celsus, advocated the use of massage in his classic work on medicine, 'De Medicina', written *c.* AD 30. He claimed that chronic pains in the head are relieved by rubbing the head itself and that a paralysed limb may be strengthened by rubbing.

Pliny the Elder (23–79 AD), the distinguished Roman naturalist, was regularly massaged to relieve his asthma and even Julius Caesar was treated daily by being pinched all over to relieve his neuralgia and headaches.

IN ANCIENT ROME MASSAGE WAS USED
TO HEAL AND RELIEVE. PAIN.

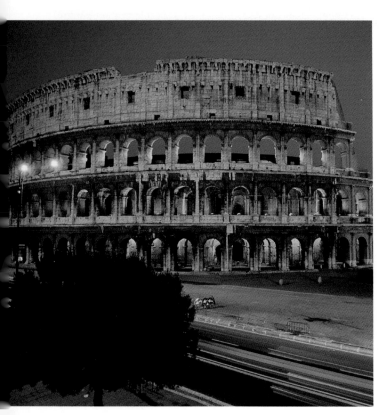

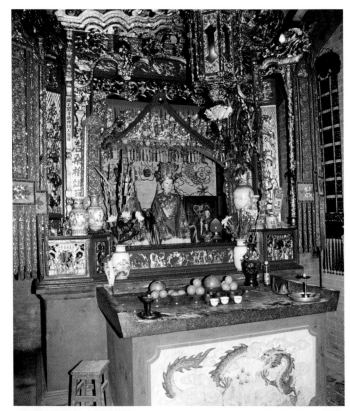

MASSAGE PLAYED AN IMPORTANT PART IN AYURVEDIC MEDICINE IN INDIA.

THE EAST

Massage was practised in China as early as 3000 BC. The Huang Ti Nei Ching Su Wen ('Yellow Emperor's Classic') was the first important medical text on Chinese medicine written around 2674 BC. The ancient Chinese technique of massage was called *amma* and is thought to have reached Japan about the 6th century AD. The Japanese called the points *tsubo*, and shiatsu, which is widely practised today, evolved from this ancient technique.

In India, Ayervedic medicine (*ayur* means life; *veda* means knowledge) is the traditional Indian system of medicine. It dates back thousands of years and includes massage amongst its principles.

EUROPE

Little evidence regarding massage can be found between the decline of the Roman Empire and the Renaissance, partly because the Catholic Church taught that pleasures of the flesh were sinful. However, the foremost early medieval philosopher and physician, Avicenna (980-1037), who was of Persian origin, wrote extensively about massage in his medical masterpiece, *The Canon of Medicine*. This was considered to be the most authoritative medical text in Europe for several centuries.

In the 16th century Ambroise Paré (*c.* 1510-1590), a French surgeon, raised awareness of the use of massage throughout the medical community.

The Swedish professor Per Henrik Ling (1776-1839) is a major figure in the history of therapeutic massage and developed the technique known as 'Swedish Massage'. He established an institute in Stockholm in 1813 for the purpose of teaching remedial massage and medical gymnastics, known as the 'Royal Gymnastic Central Institute'. In 1838, Dr Mathias Roth, an English physician who studied at Ling's institute and was author of the first English book about Swedish massage, established his own institute in London. Dr Charles Fayette Taylor, a physician from New York, who was privately taught by Roth, brought the methods to the United States in 1858.

In the beginning of the 20th century, massage therapy once again began to decline. One reason for this was that many false practitioners, taking advantage of its popularity, gave poor treatment and hurt the reputation of all practitioners.

Swedish massage spread all over the world and was widely accepted by the medical profession. In 1894 in Britain, a group of women established 'The Society of Trained Masseuses', and in 1934 it became the 'Chartered Society of Physiotherapists'. Massage formed a major part of a physiotherapy treatment until the use of electrical equipment became widespread.

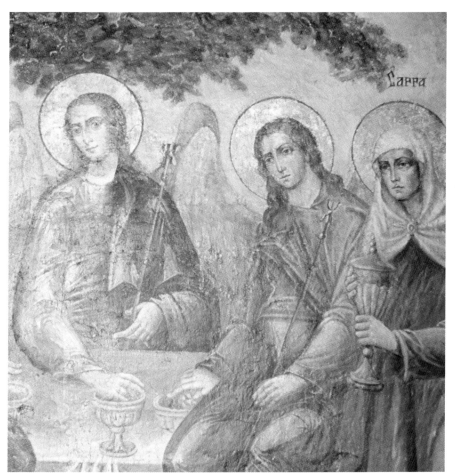

Massage enjoys an ever-growing popularity today. Therapists work alongside the medical profession in surgeries and hospitals, as well as in health clubs, beauty clinics and private practices. Many people, looking for natural, holistic ways of maintaining optimum health, are turning to massage therapy. It is a fundamental skill that I believe we should all possess.

THE CATHOLIC CHURCH CONSIDERED PLEASURES OF THE FLESH – OF ANY KIND – TO BE SINFUL.

THE BENEFITS OF MASSAGE

ALL OF US NEED TOUCH AND WE CAN ALL BENEFIT FROM MASSAGE. THE ADVANTAGES AVAILABLE TO SPECIFIC SYSTEMS OF THE BODY ARE NOTED BELOW.

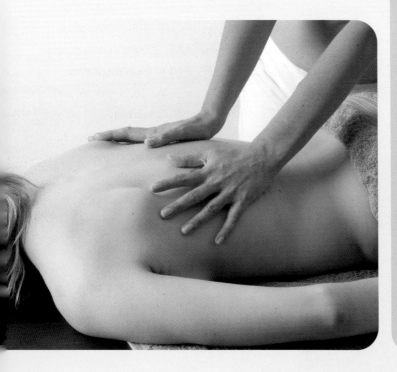

THE CIRCULATORY SYSTEM

■ The general circulation of the blood is improved since massage accelerates the flow of blood through the system. Oxygen and nutrients are brought to the cells and carbon dioxide and wastes are carried away from the cells, thus improving the functioning of the body.

■ Blood flow to the part of the body under treatment is increased. This accelerates the healing process.

■ Massage reduces high blood pressure and stress-related conditions such as rapid heartbeat (tachycardia) and disturbances in the rhythm of the heart (arrhythmia).

THE LYMPHATIC SYSTEM

■ The lymphatic system, often referred to as the body's waste disposal system, is improved. Massage accelerates the lymph flow helping to remove waste products from the system. This is particularly useful after exercise and after sustaining an injury which may be swollen, or if there is fluid retention (oedema), which needs to be dispersed by the lymphatic system. If it is not moved on it can stick to the surrounding tissues and can result in stiffness.

■ The immune system is boosted, which protects against disease.

THE GENITO-URINARY SYSTEM

■ Massage promotes activity of the kidneys, which encourages waste products to be eliminated and reduces fluid retention.

THE REPRODUCTIVE SYSTEM

■ Menstrual problems such as period pains may be helped by abdominal massage.

THE SKIN

- The texture and tone of the skin improve. Dead skin cells are removed – this process is known as desquamation – which encourages regeneration and keeps the pores open, improving skin respiration, thus enhancing texture and tone.

- The sweat and sebaceous glands are stimulated and their function is improved. Waste products are more rapidly eliminated and the sebum secreted by the sebaceous glands acts as a natural moisturiser preventing dryness and improving the elasticity of the skin.

- The colour of the skin improves. Massage increases the flow of blood to the area giving the skin a healthy vibrant glow.

THE MUSCULAR SYSTEM

- Muscular stiffness is reduced. Lactic acid and toxins that build up in over-exercised muscles can be eliminated thus reducing stiffness and fatigue.

- Pain is reduced as knots and nodules are broken down.

- Muscle spasm and cramps are relaxed.

- Muscular tone improves.

THE DIGESTIVE SYSTEM

- Massage aids the digestion of food, providing relief from conditions such as indigestion.

- Elimination is enhanced thereby alleviating and preventing conditions such as constipation.

- The muscular walls of the intestines and the abdomen are strengthened, thus encouraging digestion, absorption and elimination.

THE SKELETAL SYSTEM

- The nutrition and growth of the bones is improved.

- Stiffness of the joints is reduced and mobility is increased.

- Posture improves as tight muscles are relaxed and loose tissues are strengthened.

THE NERVOUS SYSTEM

- The nervous system may be calmed and soothed. This will reduce stress and tension and help stress-related conditions such as headaches, anxiety and insomnia.

- A stimulating massage will wake up the nervous system and help to relieve fatigue and lethargy.

THE RESPIRATORY SYSTEM

- The deeply relaxing effect of massage encourages deeper breathing and improves the efficiency of the respiratory system. Oxygen is absorbed more efficiently and carbon dioxide is removed more effectively.

- The muscles involved in respiration – namely the diaphragm and the intercostal muscles located between the ribs – are relaxed. This enables deeper, more effective respiration.

- Mucous and bronchial secretions are eliminated.

So the healing art of massage is a versatile, natural and safe therapy that can be used to treat a wide variety of common disorders and can prevent many health problems from occurring.

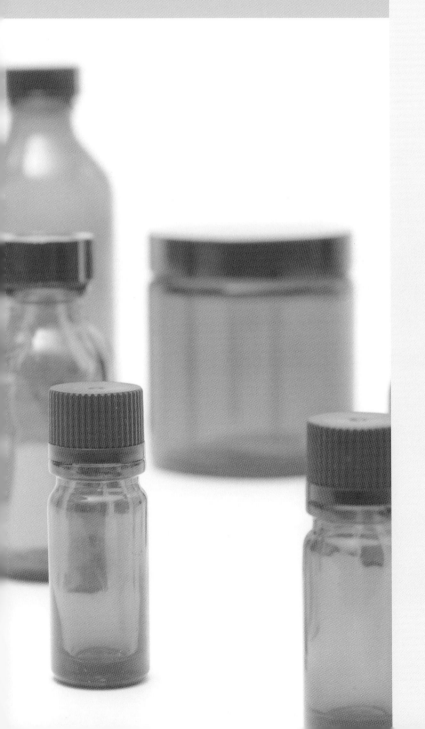

CHAPTER 1

PREPARING FOR MASSAGE

PREPARING FOR MASSAGE

WHERE TO MASSAGE

IN THEORY, A MASSAGE CAN BE CARRIED OUT ANYWHERE AND WITHOUT ANY EQUIPMENT – SOMETIMES YOU HAVE TO IMPROVISE IN PLACES THAT ARE NOT IDEAL! IN ANY ENVIRONMENT, MASSAGE CAN BRING RELIEF TO THE RECEIVER. HOWEVER, RELAXATION IS CENTRAL TO A MASSAGE AND IF YOU CAN SET THE SCENE FOR YOUR TREATMENT, THEN YOUR PARTNER WILL DERIVE MAXIMUM BENEFIT.

Here are some guidelines:

1. Make sure that there is enough space for your partner to lie down and for you to move comfortably around him or her. It is important not to feel cramped.

2. Choose a place and a time when you will not be disturbed. Take the telephone off the hook or put on the answer phone, tell your family not to disturb you and put your pets in another room if they are likely to distract you.

3. Warm up the room and make sure that it is well ventilated and draught-free. The room should be the correct temperature for your partner. Although you will get warmer as you massage, the receiver's body temperature will drop as the treatment progresses. It is not possible to relax if you are cold. Make sure that you have plenty of towels and a blanket at your disposal to cover up any areas that are not being treated and to keep the receiver warm.

4. Adjust the lighting. Glaring, overhead lighting is not conducive to relaxation. Dim the lights, use lamps or even massage by candlelight.

5. Personal touches. Add some fresh flowers to make your massage room more inviting, play some music, place some crystals in the room or use an aromatherapy burner. Essential oils for relaxation include bergamot, clary sage, chamomile, frankincense, geranium, jasmine, lavender, marjoram, neroli, rose, sandalwood and ylang ylang.

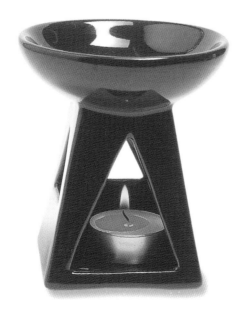

HOW TO PREPARE YOURSELF

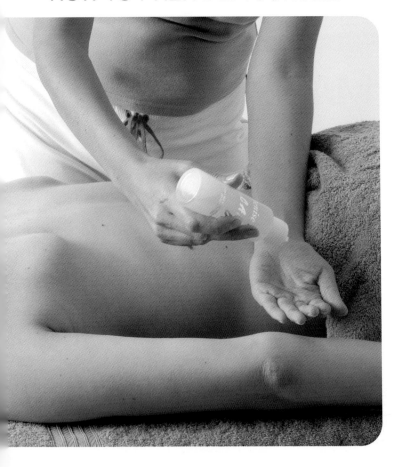

1. Wear loose, comfortable, washable clothes. It is essential that your clothes allow you to move freely around your partner. Go barefoot or wear low-healed comfortable shoes or trainers.

2. Take off jewellery especially watches, bracelets and rings with stones in which can scratch the receiver.

3. Trim your fingernails so that they do not dig into the receiver and check that your nails and hands are scrupulously clean.

4. Centre yourself. To perform massage it is important to focus solely on your massage partner. The mind is very easily distracted and can easily wander into thoughts such as 'What shall I cook tonight?', 'Have I put the rubbish out?', 'What shall I wear for work tomorrow?' Spend a few minutes prior to the massage consciously relaxing yourself. Take a few breaths and rid yourself of the stresses and strains of the day. If you feel angry or unwell then don't attempt to administer a treatment, for your energy will be depleted and negative thoughts can be picked up by the receiver.

MASSAGE SURFACES

MASSAGE COUCH

The easiest way to perform a massage is on a massage couch and if you intend to do a lot of massage it is well worth the investment. If you do decide to buy one, make sure that it has a face hole so that when the receiver is lying face down (in the prone position) the neck is in a neutral relaxed position. You should also ensure that it is the right height for you. This will prevent you from stooping down or overstretching as you work and thus protect your back from strain and injury. A good couch supplier will make a couch to suit your height and in your desired colour. The correct height for you is the height you feel comfortable to work at. However, there is a widely used and reasonably foolproof rule-of-thumb used to determine the couch height, as shown in the diagram.

MEASURING FOR A MASSAGE COUCH

To determine the correct height for your massage table stand up straight with your shoulders level, arms down by your side. Lightly clench a fist and measure from your clenched fist down to the floor. This is the correct height for you – the average height is 71 cm (28 inches).

If you do decide to purchase a massage couch, look for one that is lightweight, sturdy and portable. It is not usually practical to have a massage couch permanently erected in your home or flat! Your table should be easy to move and store. Once a massage table is folded up it looks rather like an over-sized attaché case and it can easily be put away into a corner somewhere. A portable folding massage table will either have wooden or aluminium legs – aluminium couches are slightly lighter but not quite as sturdy as wooden ones. The price of a wooden couch should start at around £225 ($350) and aluminium ones at approximately £275 ($435). Although more expensive, adjustable couches are available (priced at over £350 ($550), ask yourself how often you will need to readjust it. I would recommend opting for a basic version – extras will increase the price and are not necessary. The most expensive massage table is not necessarily the best option.

FLOOR

Don't worry if you do not have a massage couch, as you can give a very effective treatment working on the floor. To make the floor comfortable you will need adequate padding. A large piece of foam padding a couple of inches thick, a futon, folded blankets or sleeping bags are all perfectly acceptable. Ideally the massage area should extend well beyond the receiver's body. This will give you some padding to kneel on while you are giving the treatment. A massage area about 2.13 x 1.21 m (7 x 4 ft) should be big enough for most individuals. If the massage surface you have created is not big enough for you to kneel on, then you will need some cushions. Cover your massage padding with a sheet or a blanket.

A warning about beds!
Never try to massage on a bed. They are far too soft and any pressure that you apply will be absorbed by the mattress. A bed is the worst possible option to choose for a massage.

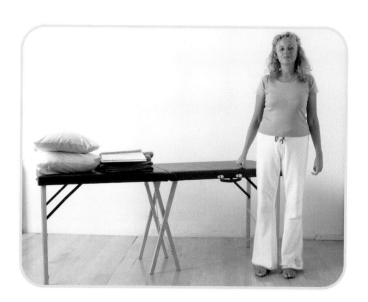

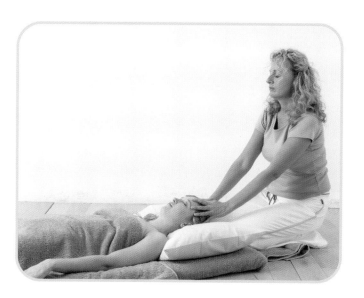

ACCESSORIES
TOWELS

It is always a good idea to keep plenty of towels on hand even if the room is warm. You will need them to cover up any area of the body that you are not working on. Towels create the feeling of trust, security and comfort, and encourage total relaxation. They also keep the body warm both before and after an area has been treated. For added relaxation, always warm your towels prior to use.

A towel should be placed on your massage couch or working area for comfort and protection. You can buy disposable paper in the form of couch roll that may be used to protect your towels from any accidental spillage of massage oil.

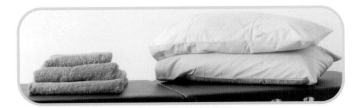

MASSAGE MEDIUMS

You will require a lubricant of some kind to carry out your massage. Oil is the most common massage medium although massage cream or talcum powder is sometimes used. You should be careful, however, to choose a pure and natural product in order to avoid an adverse skin reaction. In my opinion, the only way to massage is to use oil. This allows your hands to glide smoothly over the skin without causing any friction. Most people really like the feel of oil and if you use appropriate massage oils they are therapeutic and nourishing for the skin.

The basic oil is called a base, fixed or carrier oil, and is usually a vegetable, nut or seed oil. It should preferably be cold-pressed, unrefined and additive-free since the more highly processed the oil the less effective it will be. The use of mineral oil such as baby oil is not recommended, as it is not easily absorbed by the skin and can dry the skin and clog the pores.

Whichever carrier oil you choose, make sure that it is not too thick and heavy, otherwise it can become sticky. It is a good idea to use a lighter carrier oil such as sweet almond and

CUSHIONS AND PILLOWS

A variety of cushions and pillows will ensure the comfort of both you and the receiver.

If you are massaging the back of the body place a cushion or pillow under the neck and shoulders (unless you are working on a massage couch with a face hole ring) and one under the feet.

When treating the front of the body, place a cushion or pillow under the head and one under the knees to relax and take any strain off the lower back. You may use any other cushions you wish to create a relaxed and comfortable position for your partner. If you are working on the floor it may be necessary to place them under your own knees to avoid soreness.

perhaps add a thicker, richer oil to enhance absorption. A teaspoon of wheatgerm oil may be added to your blend to preserve it. You should also take into account the smell of the carrier oil – if you or your partner do not like the smell then there is no point in using it! You may decide to scent your carrier oil with an essential oil (see pages 18–21).

If you are working on an individual with a highly sensitive skin or with allergies you may wish to carry out a patch test. Rub a small amount of oil onto the crook of the elbow, leave for 24 hours and note if there is any reaction.

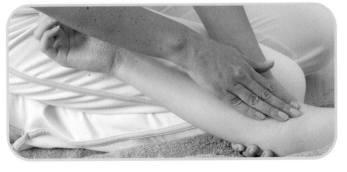

It is a good idea to carry out a patch test before using oils.

CARRIER OILS AND THEIR PROPERTIES

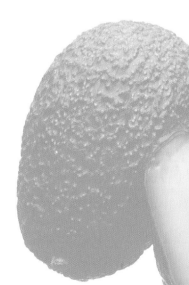

SWEET ALMOND OIL

One of the most popular base oils for massage. This light, inexpensive oil is suitable for all types of skin. It may be used on its own.

APRICOT KERNEL

Another popular oil that is suitable for all types of skin, particularly mature, inflamed, dry or sensitive skin. Apricot kernel is an excellent choice for a facial oil. It may be used alone or a small amount can be added to your primary carrier oil.

AVOCADO PEAR OIL

A rich, dark green thick carrier oil. Avocado pear is highly penetrative and is suitable for all types of skin but is particularly recommended for dry and dehydrated skin. Since it is so thick and viscous I suggest only adding a small amount to your main carrier oil.

CALENDULA

Soothing and anti-inflammatory calendula is excellent for cracked and chapped skin. It is usually added to a general base oil.

EVENING PRIMROSE OIL

An expensive base oil evening primrose oil is taken internally in capsules for a wide variety of complaints such as PMS (pre-menstrual syndrome), MS (multiple sclerosis), heart disease, psoriasis and eczema. Evening primrose oil can be used as an addition to your main base oil.

GRAPESEED

A light, inexpensive carrier oil that is almost odourless. Suitable for all skin types it may be used on its own without dilution and has no allergic effect on the skin.

PEACH KERNEL

Peach kernel oil is suitable for all skin types especially sensitive, dry and mature skins. Use it on its own as a general base oil.

JOJOBA

Jojoba oil leaves skin feeling soft and silky, yet not greasy. It is suitable for all skin types and makes an ideal facial oil. Since jojoba is relatively expensive it is normally added to a blend, but can be used alone on the face.

WHEATGERM

Wheatgerm is often added to a general oil since it is antioxidant and prevents oils from going rancid. Wheatgerm is useful for scar tissue and for preventing stretch marks. Avoid wheatgerm in cases of wheat allergy. Use it as an addition to a general blend.

Other base oils you might like to experiment with include borage seed oil, carrot oil, coconut oil, corn oil, hazelnut oil, hypericum, olive oil, peanut oil, rosehip oil, safflower oil, soybean oil and sunflower oil. Bear in mind the quality (remember cold-pressed is best), texture (not too heavy and thick) and aroma.

RECIPES FOR BASE OILS

Since they do not contain any essential oils these may be stored in 100 ml environmentally friendly high-density polythene (HDP) bottles. Don't use PVC – which releases phthalates in processing and carcinogenic dioxins when burned. HDP bottles with flip-top caps are available from reputable aromatherapy suppliers (see useful addresses at the end of the book). These containers are unbreakable and do not spill if you knock them over. However, if you have nothing else then a bowl or saucer will suffice but take care, particularly if you are working on the floor.

GENERAL BASE OIL

80 ml Sweet almond oil

5 ml Avocado oil

5 ml Peach kernel oil

5 ml Jojoba oil

5 ml Wheatgerm oil

LUXURIOUS BASE OIL

50 ml Jojoba oil

20 ml Evening primrose oil

10 ml Calendula oil

5 ml Avocado oil

5 ml Apricot kernel oil

5 ml Peach kernel oil

5 ml Wheatgerm oil

Try experimenting with your own recipes or simply use one carrier oil on its own.

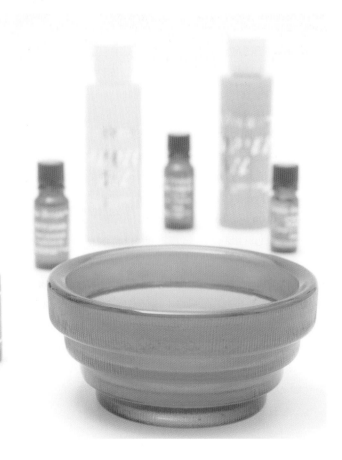

AROMATHERAPY OILS

Essential oils can greatly enhance the effects of your massage. They have a wonderful aroma and impart many therapeutic effects. Pure essential oils should always be treated with great care and used sparingly. They are highly concentrated and should never be used undiluted. Blend them with your chosen carrier oil(s) in the following dilution:

3 drops essential oil to 10 ml
  (approx 2 teaspoons of carrier oil)
6 drops essential oil to 20 ml of carrier oil
9 drops essential oil to 30 ml of carrier oil

If you are treating a small area of the body then 10 ml will be more than ample. For a complete full-body massage 20–25 ml should be sufficient, although it does depend on the size of the receiver, hairiness and condition of the skin.

A professional aromatherapist will often have a repertoire of about 60 essential oils. However, for the purposes of this book I have selected just 12 of the most common essential oils.

BERGAMOT

(Citrus bergamia)

Aroma: Light, citrus

Main properties: Astringent, balancing, uplifting

Bergamot is an excellent oil for the nerves. It lifts the mood, dispelling anxiety, irritability and depression, and energises the whole person. Bergamot is also ideal for treating acne and oily skin and hair.

Cautions: Avoid sunlight directly after treatment since bergamot increases the skin's sensitivity to sunlight.

CHAMOMILE

(Anthemis nobilis)

Aroma: Warm, sweet, fruity and apple-like

Main properties: Balancing, calming

Roman chamomile is renowned for its calming influence on all the systems of the body. It is indispensable for children and sensitive individuals. Chamomile is excellent for anger, irritability, impatience and restlessness and relives insomnia. All aches and pains such as headache, stomach ache, earache and backache will respond. Chamomile is valued for its ability to relieve inflammation and all types of skin problems.

Cautions: None

GERANIUM

(Pelargonium graveolens)

Aroma: Sweet, rose-like

Main properties: Anti-depressant, balancing

A wonderful all-round balancer for the emotions, hormones and the skin. Geranium is very healing for all skin problems and is a vital oil to use with women's problems such as PMS and the menopause. It dispels anxiety and nervous fatigue and is an excellent booster for the circulation.

Cautions: None

FRANKINCENSE

(Boswellia carterii)

Aroma: Woody, spicy

Main properties: Comforting, decongestive, rejuvenating

Frankincense is a wonderful aid for meditation since it encourages deep relaxation and enhances spiritual awareness. It is excellent for respiratory problems such as asthma, bronchitis and catarrh. Frankincense revitalises and combats ageing skin.

Cautions: None

JASMINE

(Jasminum officinale)

Aroma: Exotic, heady

Main properties: Aphrodisiac, euphoric, uplifting

A must for any love potion – couples should use jasmine for a sensual massage. Jasmine is a wonderful anti-depressant that helps to restore confidence and a positive attitude. It is also beneficial for all skin types.

Cautions: None

LAVENDER

(Lavendula augustifolia/vera/officinalis)

Aroma: Sweet, floral

Main properties: Balancing, calming, pain-relieving, healing

One of the most versatile essential oils – every home should have a bottle of lavender. If you only buy one oil get this one! Lavender has a calming effect on the nerves relieving anxiety, tension, and all stress-related problems such as headaches, palpitations and insomnia. Lavender is excellent for all aches and pains, cuts and burns, digestive disorders, menstrual problems and skin care. It also boosts the immune system.

Cautions: None

LEMON

(Citrus limonum)

Aroma: Clean, fruity, refreshing

Main properties: Antiseptic, detoxifying

A marvellous pick-me-up, lemon helps to speed up recovery and assists concentration and clear thinking. Lemon is indicated for slimming, detoxification, cellulite, fluid retention and wrinkles, and is an excellent overall tonic.

Cautions: Avoid strong sunlight immediately after treatment.

NEROLI

(Citrus aurantium)

Aroma: Floral, haunting

Main properties: Anti-depressant, aphrodisiac, uplifting

The beautiful aroma of neroli is invaluable for all emotional problems. It lifts depression and induces peace and a sense of euphoria. Neroli is excellent for sexual problems such as impotence and frigidity. It is highly recommended for all skin types since it is regenerative.

Cautions: None

ROSE OTTO

(Rosa damascena)

Aroma: Exquisite, heady, intoxicating

Main properties: Balancing, calming, tonic

A wonderful oil that helps to dispel depression, tension and feelings of inadequacy. Rose is a must for all women's problems and skin care. It also helps constipation.

Cautions: None

ROSEMARY

(Rosmarinus officinalis)

Aroma: Clean, strong, herby

Main properties: Pain-relieving, tonic

Rosemary is a physical as well as a mental stimulant aiding mental clarity, concentration and dispelling fatigue. It is used to treat all muscular aches and pains, bringing relief and inducing muscle tone. Rosemary is a cleansing oil, making it beneficial for cellulite and any digestive problems if detoxification is required.

Cautions: Do not use extensively on epileptics

SANDALWOOD

(Santalum album)

Aroma: Sweet, warm, lingering

Main properties: Aphrodisiac, calming, peaceful

Sandalwood is excellent for the nervous system inducing a deep sense of relaxation and dispelling anxiety. It is marvellous for all skin types especially dry, dehydrated and mature skin.

Cautions: None

YLANG YLANG

(Canaga odorata)

Aroma: Exotic, heady, sweet

Main properties: Aphrodisiac, euphoric, sedative

Ylang ylang is used extensively for nervous problems since it allays anxiety and depression. It reduces high blood pressure and calms palpitation. Ylang ylang is suitable for all types of skin.

Cautions: None

These essential oils may be used singly blended in a carrier oil, or you may like to try one of the following recipes or even formulate your own.

RECIPES FOR AROMATHERAPY BLENDS

Dilute the following in 20 ml carrier oil.

RELAXING BLEND

GERANIUM 2 DROPS

LAVENDER 2 DROPS

SANDALWOOD 2 DROPS

STIMULATING BLEND

LEMON 3 DROPS

ROSEMARY 3 DROPS

UPLIFTING BLEND

BERGAMOT 2 DROPS

GERANIUM 2 DROPS

JASMINE 2 DROPS

WOMEN'S BLEND

CHAMOMILE 2 DROPS

GERANIUM 3 DROPS

ROSE 3 DROPS

APHRODISIAC BLEND

JASMINE 2 DROPS

NEROLI 2 DROPS

SANDALWOOD 2 DROPS

HEAVENLY BLEND

FRANKINCENSE 2 DROPS

NEROLI 2 DROPS

ROSE 1 DROP

INSOMNIA BLEND

CHAMOMILE 2 DROPS

LAVENDER 2 DROPS

NEROLI 2 DROPS

EXOTIC BLEND

FRANKINCENSE 2 DROPS

SANDALWOOD 2 DROPS

YLANG YLANG 2 DROPS

APPLYING THE OIL

It is important to apply the oil properly for best results. Too little oil could leave the skin irritated and sore and even cause a rash. A hairy chest, back or leg will certainly require extra oil – you do not want to irritate the hair follicles or pull the hair as you massage over the area. Too much oil and you will find it very difficult to carry out the deeper massage movements such as friction. Your hands will slip and slide over the skin and the receiver will feel sticky and uncomfortable when they put their clothes on. Therefore, it is best to apply the oil little and often.

1. Never pour oil directly from the bottle onto the receiver's body. It is not a pleasant sensation particularly if you have not warmed the oil prior to the treatment. If you wish, the oil can be warmed by placing it on top of a radiator or by placing it in a jug of warm water. First dispense a small amount of oil – about half a teaspoon – into the palm of one of your hands.

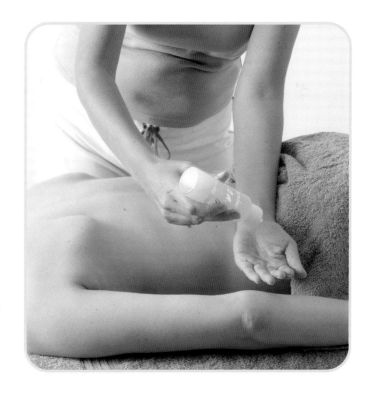

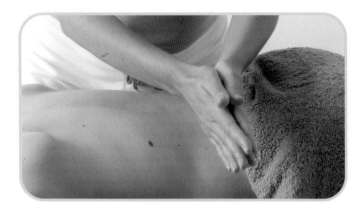

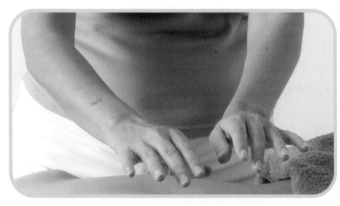

2. Then rub your hands briskly together to warm both the oil and your hands. Make sure that the hand into which you are dispensing the oil is slightly by the side of your massage partner's body rather than directly over it. If you do spill a few drops of oil they will not fall directly onto the receiver. You can always apply more oil if you need it. If you do put too much oil on then you can remove the excess with your forearms.

3. After rubbing your palms together, allow your hands to float slowly down onto the part of the body on which you are going to work and allow them to rest there for a few moments. Once you have established this initial contact, begin to apply the oil with the palms of both hands using stroking movements. This initial contact is important: do not thrust your hands down suddenly onto the receiver's back, as this can be a shock to his or her system.

Once you have established contact it is vital to maintain it. Breaking contact with your partner destroys the continuity and harmony of the treatment. Therefore, always try to have at least one hand on the receiver throughout the massage.

Take care where you put your bottle of oil. Put it somewhere that you can find it easily but in a place where it will not get knocked over.

DOS AND DON'TS OF OILING

DO

- Apply oil little and often.
- Warm the oil prior to the treatment.
- Warm your hands and the oil by briskly, rubbing them together.
- Use more oil for a hairy body.
- Establish your initial contact gently and slowly.

DON'T

- Pour the oil directly onto the receiver's body.
- Allow drops of oil to drip onto the receiver.
- Break contact during the treatment.

POSTURE

YOU SHOULD ALWAYS PAY ATTENTION TO YOUR POSTURE WHETHER YOU ARE WORKING AT A TABLE, SITTING, OR KNEELING ON THE FLOOR, AND PARTICULARLY IF YOU ARE PERFORMING LOTS OF MASSAGES.

Many people who suffer with muscle and joint problems do so because of incorrect posture. If your posture is incorrect you can strain your own body and then you will be the one who needs a massage! If you feel uncomfortable the receiver will become aware of your discomfort since your movements will not flow easily and freely.

WORKING AT A MASSAGE COUCH

If you are working on a couch this helps to eliminate some of the bending and puts less strain on your own body. However, you should still take note of the following guidelines:

- Keep your back straight.
- Keep your knees slightly bent – bending your knees rather than your back eliminates a great deal of potential strain in your lower back.
- Keep your weight evenly distributed between both legs.
- Keep your feet apart with your toes pointing out at approximately 45°.

- Keep your neck and shoulders relaxed.
- Keep your wrists and hands supple and relaxed.
- Keep the neck straight – do not drop the head forward when looking down.
- Keep the jaw relaxed.
- Stand close to the couch to avoid overreaching.
- Move around the couch whenever necessary ensuring that you do not lose contact with the receiver.
- Use your whole body to massage – not just your hands.

CORRECT POSTURE (I)

Stand with your feet well apart, knees bent, back straight with no tension in the arms, neck or shoulders. Ensure that your weight is evenly distributed through the legs.

CORRECT POSTURE (II)
THE LUNGE POSITION.

Stand at the side of the couch, feet apart, one in front of the other. Keep the back leg fairly straight but not rigid and the front leg slightly bent and try shifting your body weight forward onto the front leg. This position allows you to use the weight of your body to apply pressure.

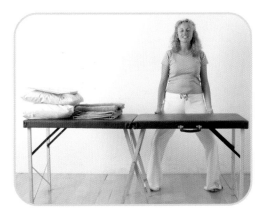

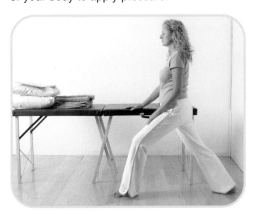

CONTRAINDICATIONS: WHEN NOT TO MASSAGE

Although massage is one of the safest therapies available, there are some occasions when it is not appropriate to massage or caution needs to be exercised. Therefore, prior to a massage treatment check that none of the following conditions exist. If you are in any doubt then always seek the advice of a medically qualified doctor.

FEVER

A high temperature indicates that the body is fighting off toxins. Massage releases toxins and the body already has enough to cope with.

INFECTIOUS AND CONTAGIOUS DISEASES

You do not wish to contract the disease yourself or pass it on to others, particularly illnesses that affect the skin such as chicken pox, scabies and impetigo.

THROMBO-PHLEBITIS

A thrombus is a blood clot which if dislodged could result in a fatal stroke or a heart attack. Therefore, it is extremely dangerous to massage if someone has thrombosis.

RECENT OPERATIONS OR SCARS

Massage could open up a recent scar and even cause an infection. Depending on whether the operation is a major or a minor one there will be varying degrees of scarring. It is always best for your massage partner to check with his or her doctor.

AREAS OF INFLAMMATION

Inflammation may occur after a joint sprain or muscle strain. There may also be inflammation of an internal organ such as nephritis (inflammation of the kidney). Massage over an inflamed area can cause further inflammation. The signs of inflammation include heat, swelling, redness and pain.

VARICOSE VEINS

Pressure can produce further damage to the walls of the blood vessels as well as cause discomfort. Stroking movements over the area are acceptable and may ease the pressure off the vein and aid repair. Deeper movements such as friction are not advisable.

PREGNANCY

Massage during pregnancy can be very beneficial helping to ease many minor complaints. Indeed, many pregnant women instinctively massage their own abdomen. However, special care should be taken over the abdomen during the first three months particularly if there is a risk of miscarriage. If there is any doubt consult the doctor.

SKIN PROBLEMS

It is common sense to avoid a cut, abrasion, bite, sunburn etc, as it would be painful.

BROKEN BONES

It should be a matter of common sense not to massage if a bone is broken or assumed to be broken. Medical help should always be sought. In any event, it would cause so much pain that the receiver would not tolerate it!

UNDIAGNOSED LUMPS, BUMPS, MOLES

These should always be checked by a medically qualified doctor.

OSTEOPOROSIS

If the receiver has brittle bones then only very gentle movements should be used. In severe cases check it out with the doctor.

ALCOHOL OR DRUGS

It is common sense not to massage someone heavily under the influence of drugs or alcohol.

CANCER/TUMOURS

Do not massage over the site of a tumour. Cancer patients derive great comfort from massage, and oncology (cancer) units often have massage therapists. However, you should never massage directly over the site of a tumour, any radiotherapy site or skin cancer.

HEART PROBLEMS

Many heart problems such as high blood pressure can be helped enormously with massage. With severe cardiovascular problems, however, it is always best to check with a doctor.

DIABETES

Diabetes is not a contraindication, but one should bear in mind that the condition can affect the peripheral circulation, especially in the feet. This can cause the skin to be thinner and more susceptible to bruising. If the nerves are affected there may be a loss of sensory function and patients will be unable to give you accurate information regarding pressure. Do not press too hard!

MASSAGE IS GENERALLY VERY SAFE, BUT IF IN DOUBT CONSULT A MEDICAL DOCTOR.

CHAPTER 2

BASIC TECHNIQUES

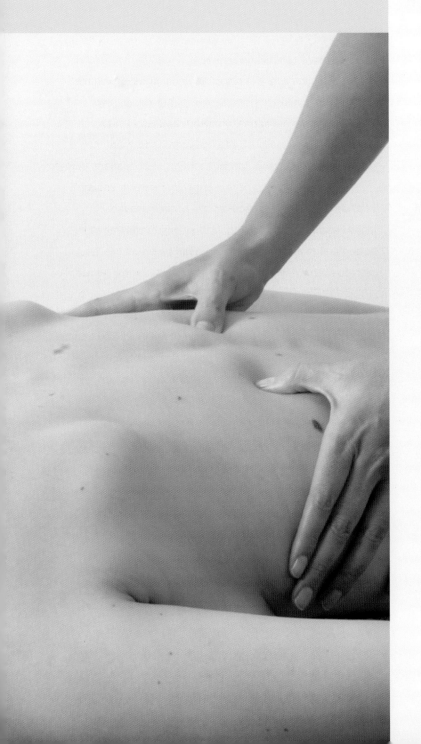

BASIC TECHNIQUES

IN THIS SECTION YOU WILL FIND DETAILED DESCRIPTIONS AND PHOTOGRAPHS OF THE PRINCIPAL TECHNIQUES USED IN MASSAGE. THEY ARE THE FUNDAMENTAL MOVEMENTS FROM WHICH YOU WILL DEVELOP YOUR OWN PERSONAL MASSAGE STYLE. LET YOUR HANDS GUIDE YOU AND TRY TO BE SPONTANEOUS. HERE ARE A FEW GUIDELINES.

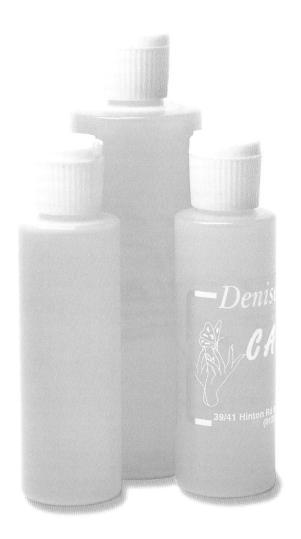

- Don't try to do too much or learn too much at once. It is not necessary to learn the entire massage repertoire in a single session! Start by practising a few massage strokes and build up gradually. In the beginning if you have never massaged before you may find it a little tiring but it will soon become effortless.

- Don't worry if your movements feel a little clumsy or awkward at first. It may be because you are trying too hard. We all have a natural ability to massage and you will be amazed at how quickly your massage movements begin to flow.

- Ask your massage partner for feedback. What is the pressure like – too hard, too light or just right? Are the movements too fast or too slow? Does your massage partner feel comfortable and relaxed, is he or she warm enough? When you first start practising the basic massage techniques, feedback is invaluable. As you become more familiar, relaxed and confident you will find that the communication between you becomes more non-verbal. Your hands will pick up most of the information that you need and you will be able to tune into the amount of pressure and speed required almost instinctively. This is excellent, for the less said during a massage the better. It is most powerful and deeply healing when it is performed in silence – words can be a distraction.

- Try practising the movements on yourself or even better ask your partner to perform them on you. There is no better way to learn massage than to experience it yourself.

ENJOY IT!

EFFLEURAGE

The word 'effleurage' is derived from the French *effleurer* which means to touch or stroke lightly. Effleurage is exactly this – the stroking movement of massage. It is performed at the very beginning of a massage and serves initially to distribute the massage medium. Stroking is the first contact with the massage partner and it enables him or her to become relaxed and accustomed to your touch. It is through soothing effleurage that a sense of trust and rapport is established between you and the receiver. Effleurage gives you the opportunity to 'sense' any problem areas. Stroking may be performed between techniques since it provides a link from one movement to the next. Effleurage prepares the body for deeper movements and at the end of a massage helps to drain away any toxins that have been released by the deeper techniques.

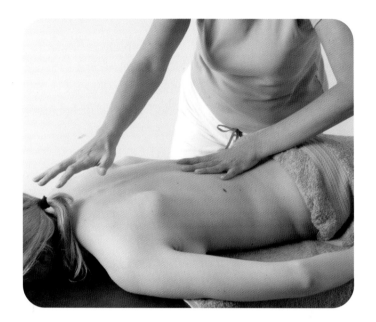

WHAT ARE ITS THERAPEUTIC EFFECTS?

- Effleurage accustoms the receiver to your touch and enables you to spread the massage oil.
- If performed slowly it soothes the nerves, deeply relaxing the receiver. Effleurage is invaluable for anxiety, tension, anger and irritability. Stroking techniques can relieve insomnia and other stress-related disorders such as headaches.
- Effleurage warms up the tissue bringing fresh blood to the area and improving the circulation.
- Stroking encourages the flow of lymph relieving congestion and flushing away any toxins.

- The nutrition of the skin is improved since effleurage helps to desquamate (remove dead skin cells) encouraging new cell growth and hence fresh, glowing skin.
- When performed quickly effleurage stimulates the nervous system making one feel energised and revitalised.
- Stroking helps to release tension from the muscles as it gently loosens the adhered fibres.
- Effleurage enables you to detect any areas that may feel tighter, tenser or harder than others.

HOW TO DO IT

Effleurage is performed with the palms of either one or both hands when working over a large area. The pads of the fingers or thumbs may be employed if a small area such as the wrist is to be treated. Stroking is always smooth and rhythmic rather than abrupt and jerky. The hands stay very relaxed and mould to the contours of the body. As much of the hands as possible should remain in contact with the body, with the pressure focused through the heels of the palms rather than the fingers. The hands stay in contact with the body at all times so that there is no break in the massage.

Pressure is usually applied towards the heart or in the direction of the underlying muscle fibres. In other words up the back, up the arms and legs and down the neck and shoulders. The pressure is applied on the upward stroke and the hands return to their starting point with no pressure whatsoever.

Sometimes effleurage may be performed in a centripetal direction – i.e. in a circle moving towards the centre. You should use your whole body not just your hands to perform effleurage or indeed any other massage technique.

If you wish to apply deeper pressure simply place one hand on top of the other. You are using a smaller area of contact to achieve a deeper stroke. To work even more deeply into the tissues a smaller contact point such as the pads of the thumb or fingers may be used.

LETS PRACTISE!

When practising these techniques pour a small amount of oil onto one of your hands and rub your palms briskly together to warm the oil. Remember it is best to apply the oil little and often to avoid breaking contact. Rest a part of your forearm lightly against the receiver's body as you disperse the oil.

1. EFFLEURAGE THE BACK

A. LONG STROKING (BOTH HANDS)

POSITION

At the side of the receiver.

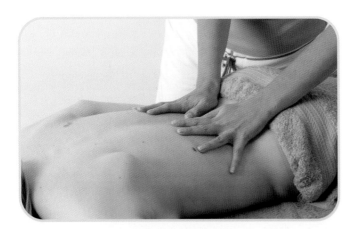

1. Place both hands, flat, on either side of the spine, at the bottom of the back. Your fingers should face upwards.

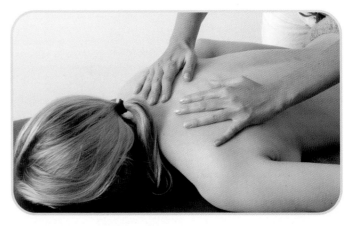

2. Stroke up the entire length of the back and across the shoulders. Maintain a firm pressure and use your body weight.

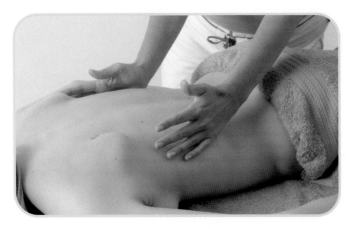

3. Allow your hands to glide back to their starting point, lightly skimming across the skin using no pressure whatsoever.

Repeat your effleurage movements many times, maintaining an even rhythm. Ensure that your hands stay in contact with the body at all times and allow them to mould to the contours of the back. These strokes should feel like one continuous massage movement. There should be no jerkiness whatsoever. To heighten sensitivity close your eyes as you effleurage.

B. LONG STROKING (ALTERNATE HANDS)

POSITION

At the side of the receiver.

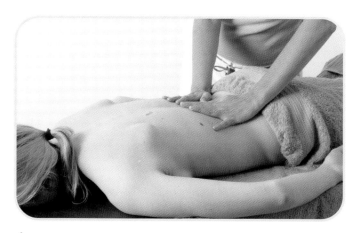

1. Place both hands palms downwards on the lower back.

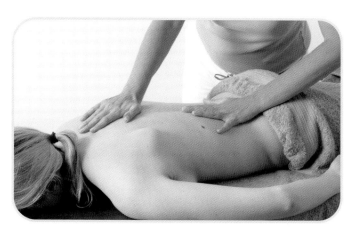

2. Effleurage firmly up the back and over the shoulder with one hand only and allow it to glide back with no pressure.

3. As the first hand completes the movement, repeat the movement with your other hand on the other side of the back. Maintain a smooth and even rhythm as you repeat these movements many times, experimenting with different speeds and pressures.

C. CIRCULAR STROKING

POSITION

At the side of the receiver.

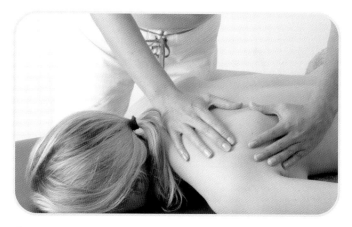

1. Place the palms of both hands on the opposite side of the body around the shoulder blade.

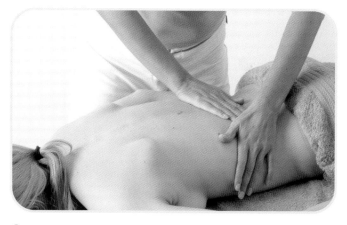

2. Make large stroking movements around the shoulder blade in a circular motion with one hand following the other. As you perform the circles your hands will cross over. Even though you will have to lift one hand over the other make sure that one hand always has contact with the body.

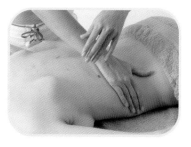

3. Repeat the circular stroking down the body towards the buttocks area. Then work back up the body towards the neck.

D. DOUBLE-HANDED CIRCULAR STROKING

POSITION

At the side of the receiver.

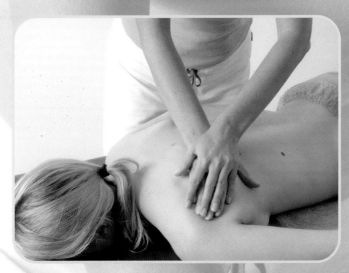

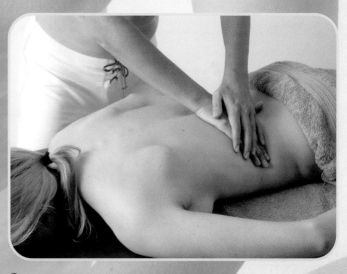

1. Put one hand flat on top of the other and place your hands on the opposite side of the body. Make large outward circular movements around the scapula.

2. Continue the reinforced stroking working down towards the buttocks and then back up again.

By putting one hand on top of the other with the same effort you will find you can achieve a much deeper pressure.

E. CAT STROKING

1. Place the whole of the palm of one hand at the base of the receiver's neck. Stroke slowly down the body using very little pressure. As one hand reaches the buttocks as you gently lift it off, repeat the movement with the other hand. Make sure that at no time contact is lost with the receiver. It should feel like one continuous movement.

POSITION

At the side of the receiver.

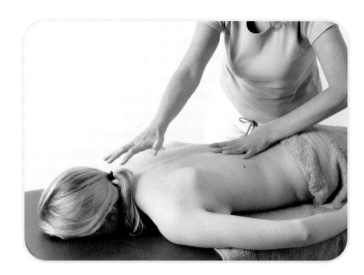

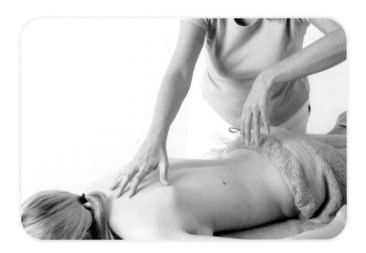

2. As a variation, repeat the same technique using just the fingertips of your hands so that they are barely touching the skin.

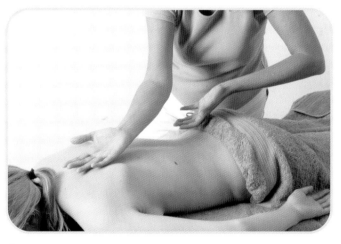

3. As another variation repeat this technique using the back of the hands.

Cat stroking movements are very soothing and deeply relaxing and are perfect to use as a finishing touch after you have completed a massage of a part of the body.

2. EFFLEURAGE THE BACK OF THE LEG

A. BOTH HANDS

POSITION

At the side of the receiver.

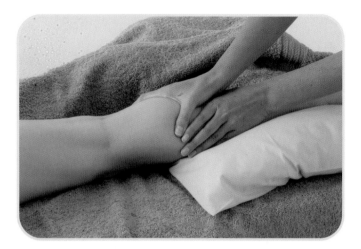

1. Place both hands, palms down, in a V-shape just above the heel. One hand should be just above the other.

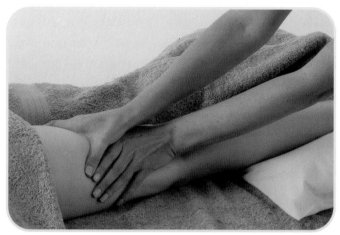

2. Stroke firmly up the calf and thigh muscles, moulding your hands to the contours of the leg. Apply very little pressure to the back of the knee since it is a delicate area.

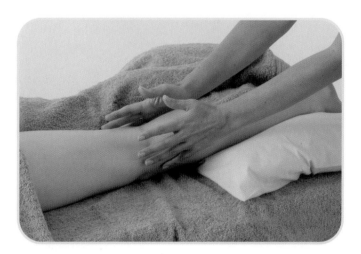

3. As your hands reach the top of the thigh allow them to separate and glide them back down the sides of the leg using virtually no pressure whatsoever. Repeat these strokes many times, gradually increasing the pressure.

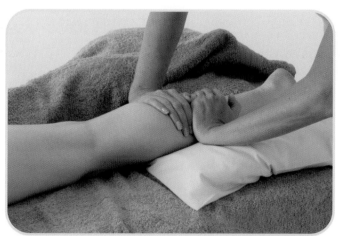

4. As a variation, place one hand across the back of the ankle with the fingertips pointing in one direction and your other hand just above with fingertips pointing in the other direction. Effleurage up the leg, taking care over the back of the knee, fan your hands out at the top of the thigh just as you did previously and allow your hands to glide gently back to your starting point. Repeat this movement many times.

B. ALTERNATE HANDS

1. Cup one hand in a V-shape over the back of the ankle. Use firm pressure to stroke smoothly up the back of the leg going more lightly over the back of the knee. As your first hand reaches the top of the thigh gently lift it off and repeat the movement with the other hand. Ensure that contact is never broken.

POSITION
At the side of the receiver.

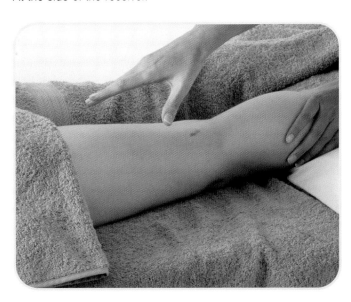

C. DOUBLE HANDED

POSITION
At the side of the receiver.

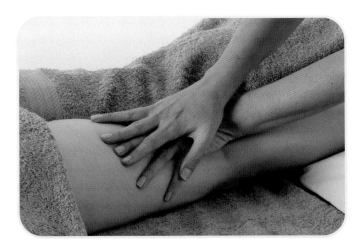

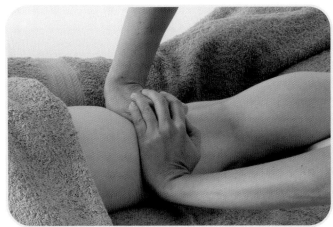

1. Place one hand palm downwards over the ankle and place your other hand on top of it. Your fingertips should be pointing upwards. Move both hands together up the leg, going more lightly over the back of the knee. Separate your hands at the top of the thigh and return back down the leg with a feather-light touch.

2. As a variation cup, one hand over the back of the ankle, fingers pointing in one direction and the other hand on top of it with fingertips pointing in the other direction.

PETRISSAGE

The word 'petrissage' is derived from the French *pétrir* which means to knead (bread or dough) and to mould or shape (clay). If you like to work with clay or make your own bread you will find this technique very easy!

Petrissage is a deeper technique and should be employed only after the tissues have been warmed up and prepared by effleurage. The muscular tissue is lifted and gently moved away from the underlying structure, squeezed and then released. It is particularly suitable for large muscle groups such as the thighs, buttocks, sides of the abdomen, upper arms and across the top of the shoulders. It would not be suitable for delicate or bony areas such as the face. There are a variety of petrissage movements including picking-up, squeezing, rolling, wringing and kneading. Petrissage may be performed either gently or vigorously to produce a soothing or a stimulating effect.

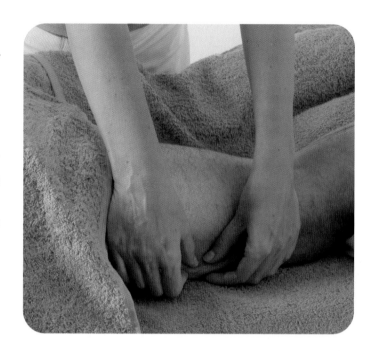

WHAT ARE ITS THERAPEUTIC EFFECTS?

- Petrissage brings an increased blood supply to the muscles being worked on. It encourages fresh nutrients and oxygen to be delivered to the area.
- It is decongestive, assisting the removal of toxins from the deeper tissues and encouraging their elimination.
- Since petrissage stretches the muscular tissue and prevents the build up of toxins like lactic acid it is excellent for preventing stiffness in muscles following exercise.

- It is tremendous for softening adhesions and relieving muscle spasms.
- Petrissage is of enormous value in the treatment of obesity. It helps to break down fatty deposits, for instance around the thighs and buttocks, if it is performed vigorously. The fatty tissue is softened by the petrissage allowing the fatty deposits to be absorbed by the lymphatics.
- The tone of the muscles also improves with the application of petrissage.

HOW TO DO IT

PICKING UP

Picking up is performed by slowly and carefully grasping the muscle with either one or both hands and then lifting and stretching the muscle away from the bone as far as possible. The tissues are then released, whilst your hands remain in contact, and are allowed to return to their resting position. Thus the muscle is alternately lifted and relaxed. It is very important to keep the thumbs well outstretched and to ensure that the palm plays a major part in the lifting. This will eliminate the possibility of nipping and pinching the flesh.

SQUEEZING

Squeezing naturally follows on as the second movement of petrissage. After you have picked up the muscle the tissues are gently squeezed and released. So the muscle is lifted, gently squeezed and then released to cleanse the deeper tissues of toxins.

ROLLING

Rolling is the third petrissage movement since it follows on from the two previous movements. The muscle mass is picked up, squeezed and then can be rolled transversely in both directions. The tissues are rolled by moving the thumbs towards the fingers and then by working the fingers towards the thumbs.

When performing picking up, and rolling ensure that you are moving the muscle tissue and not merely the skin. If only the skin is moved the technique is known as 'skin rolling'.

WRINGING

In this technique the muscle is literally 'wrung out' more or less like the action that is used when wringing out a chamois leather. Use alternate hands to pick up the muscle and wring it out. It is like picking up with a twist.

This is an excellent movement for helping to release muscle spasms. It can be performed slowly to soothe and relax or quickly and vigorously to create a stimulating effect. A steady rhythm should be established whether this movement is performed quickly or slowly.

KNEADING

Kneading is rather similar to wringing. However, instead of lifting the muscles as in all the other petrissage techniques, a downwards pressure is applied. Pressure is applied towards the body rather than away from it.

LETS PRACTISE!

When practising petrissage the amount of oil that you use is crucial. If you use too little oil your hands will not be able to flow and you could pinch the skin. If you use too much your hands will slide around and it will be very difficult to pick up any muscle! Always effleurage the area thoroughly prior to practising the petrissage.

1. PICKING UP (SQUEEZING) THE INNER THIGH/CALF

POSITION
At the side of the receiver, facing the leg to be treated.

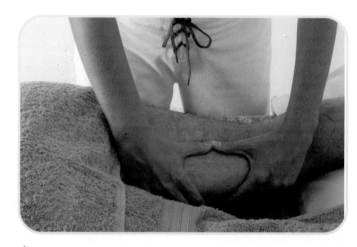

1. Place both hands, flat on the inside of the thigh. Your thumbs should be well outstretched.

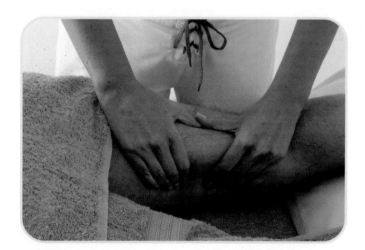

2. Gently and slowly lift the muscle away from the bone. Repeat several times. Now gently pick up and squeeze the muscle and then release it. Use the whole of your hands especially the palms and ensure that you are working on the muscle and not just the skin. Repeat the picking up and squeezing many times.

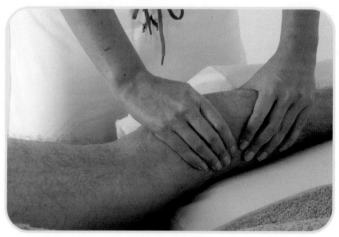

3. Now try picking up and picking up and squeezing on the calf muscles.

2. ROLLING THE OUTER THIGH/CALF

POSITION

At the side of the receiver but on the opposite side of the leg to be treated.

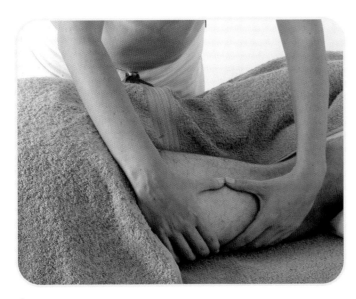

1. You will be treating the leg furthest away from you. Place both hands, flat on the outer thigh muscles.

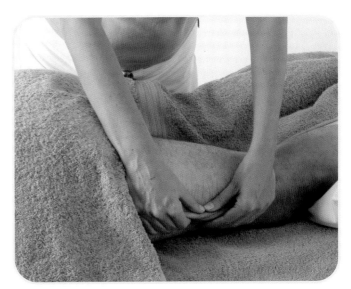

2. Pick up the muscle and roll the thumbs towards the fingers. Repeat several times.

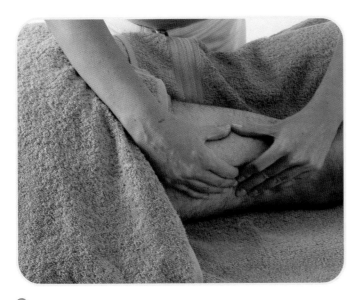

3. Now pick up the muscle and use your fingers to roll the muscle towards your thumbs. Remember to ensure you roll the muscle and not just the skin.

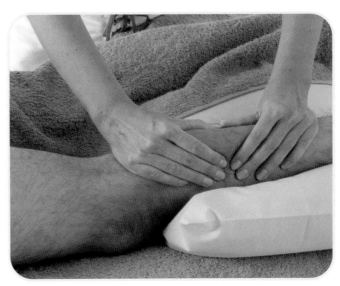

4. Repeat the rolling action on the calf muscles, maintaining an even and steady rhythm.

3. WRINGING THE SIDES OF THE BACK/ACROSS THE SHOULDERS

POSITION

On the opposite side of the part of the body to be treated.

1. Place both hands, flat down, on the muscles at the side of the torso.

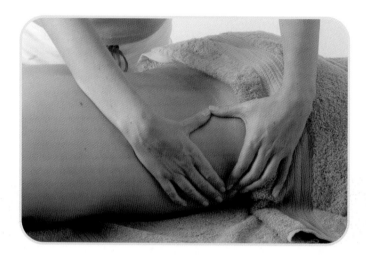

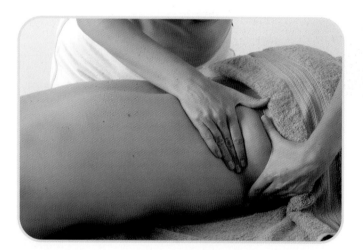

2. Use alternate hands to pick up and wring the muscles, trying to create a similar action to wringing out a chamois leather. Your movements should be firm and rhythmic with no pinching.

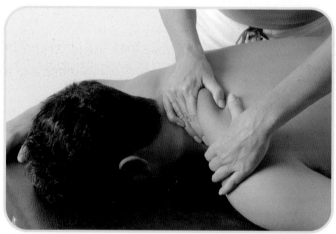

3. Now try the technique of wringing over the tops of the shoulders. If this area is very tense, then perform some picking up and squeezing first to loosen up and prepare the muscle for wringing.

4. KNEADING THE ABDOMEN/ARMS

Kneading the abdomen improves the tone of the abdominal muscles and helps to alleviate digestive problems such as constipation. The abdominal muscles need to be relaxed so no talking or laughing when practising this technique!

POSITION

At the side of the receiver's abdomen.

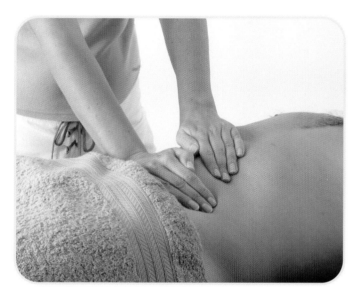 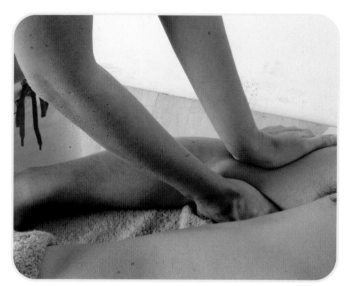

1. Place one or both hands, palms downwards, flat on the abdominal area. Apply downward pressure (NOT a 'lifting' action as in the other petrissage movements) to perform kneading movements with the hands moving in the same or in opposite directions. The pressure is made alternately between the heel of the hand and the fingers.

2. To perform kneading on a limb, the hands are placed on alternate sides of it. Place the palm of one hand flat down on the front of the arm and the palm of the other hand on the back of the arm. Press the tissues between your hands and perform large circular movements with your hands working in different directions. Work the entire upper arm in this way.

FRICTION

The word 'friction' is derived from the Latin *fricare* which means to rub. It is a deep technique particularly useful for loosening and breaking up knots, nodules and old scar tissue. Friction is used mostly near bones to move the muscle mass against the bone. It is excellent for use around joints. It is a very powerful and stimulating technique, and sensitivity is required to determine just the right amount of pressure.

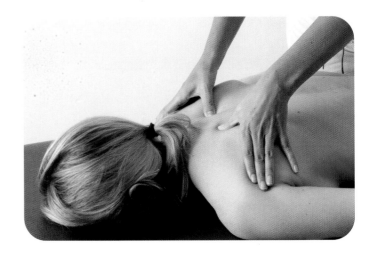

WHAT ARE ITS THERAPEUTIC EFFECTS?

- Friction breaks up adhesions and nodules.
- Friction breaks down fatty deposits.
- It accelerates the flow of blood to the area under treatment thus raising the temperature.
- Friction helps to eliminate accumulated waste products.
- It loosens up stiff joints increasing circulation and releasing fibrous adhesions.

- Friction helps to break down old scar tissue – it should not be used on or around recent scar tissue.
- It can provide analgesia (pain relief).
- Friction stimulates the nerves and improves and maintains the nutrition and the function of the nerves.

HOW TO DO IT

Friction is performed most often with the pads of thumbs or fingers. However, pressure may be applied with the knuckles, the heel of the hand or even the elbows. It consists of small circular movements whereby the muscle is moved against the bone. Since it is a pressure movement it is necessary to stand directly over the area to be treated. The elbow may be stiffened in order to penetrate even more deeply into the tissues.

LETS PRACTISE!

Since friction is a deep technique, it is important to prepare the area before practice with some effleurage movements. Take care not to use too much oil, otherwise your thumbs will slip and slide around and it will be difficult to palpate any problem areas. After you have frictioned an area always make sure that you effleurage afterwards to soothe the area and drain away any toxins.

1. FRICTION THE BACK

POSITION
At the side of the receiver directly over the part to be treated.

1. Place both hands either side of the spine and put the pads of your thumbs in the dimples at the base of the spine.

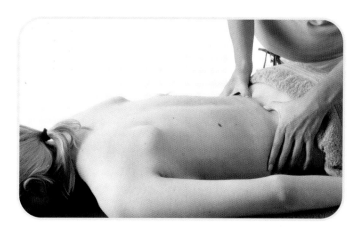

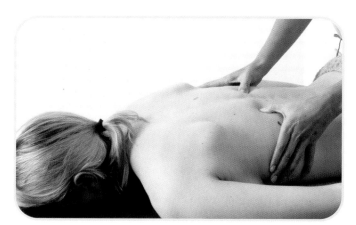

2. Perform small, deep circular friction movements, gradually working from the dimples up towards the base of the neck. As your thumbs are unaccustomed to performing friction they may ache to begin with, but they will soon adapt. To increase the pressure and reach the deeper tissues, use your body weight to lean into the movement. You may also try stiffening the elbows to achieve more pressure.

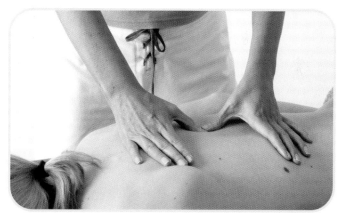

3. If you find a nodule, friction over the area with the balls of your thumbs. Friction can be uncomfortable but most people describe it as a 'good pain'. It should not be too forceful, however, and friction may only be applied for a short period at a time – approximately a minute. You may return to the same area later on in the massage session but try not to overdo it or the tissues can become irritated.

For a deeper pressure, place one thumb on top of the other, with the fingers splayed out to give support and control, and move your thumbs in a circular direction.

The knuckles may also be used to treat an area with deep friction. Make a fist and place it onto a knotty area and circle over it slowly and deeply.

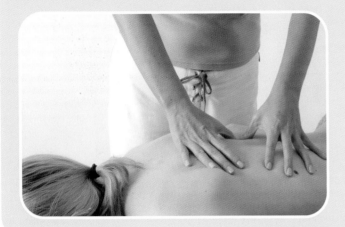
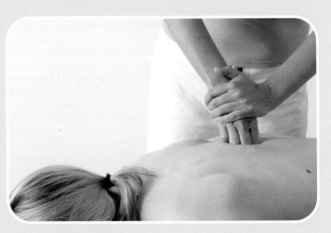

2. FRICTION AROUND THE PATELLA (KNEECAP)

POSITION

At the side of the receiver facing the knee you wish to treat.

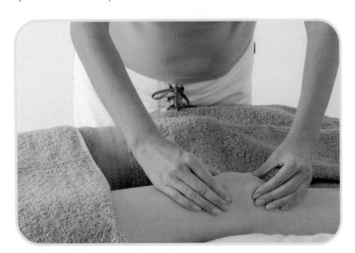
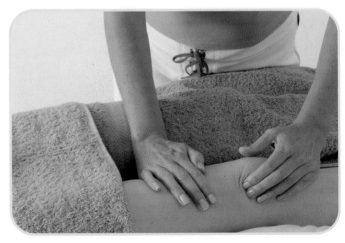

1. Place your thumbs and index fingers around the patella. The kneecap is much smaller than you think – you will be able to feel the edges of the bone if you are in the right position.

2. Friction all around the kneecap paying extra special attention to any troublesome areas.

PERCUSSION/TAPOTEMENT

The word 'percussion' is derived from the Latin *percutere* which means to hit. Tapotement is a stimulating, invigorating technique that involves striking the tissues with alternate hands in rapid succession in different ways. Various parts of the hands are used to perform percussion movements: the edge of the hands, the palms and the fists. The secret of tapotement lies in the flexibility of the wrists, since this is where the action comes from, rather than the elbows or shoulders.

Percussion movements should only be performed over the larger muscle areas of the body such as the thighs. It is never performed over bony prominences such as the shins. As tapotement is stimulating it is used in massages where a vigorous approach is required. It is invaluable for use on athletes prior to an event. However, if relaxation is the primary aim it may not be appropriate to perform it!

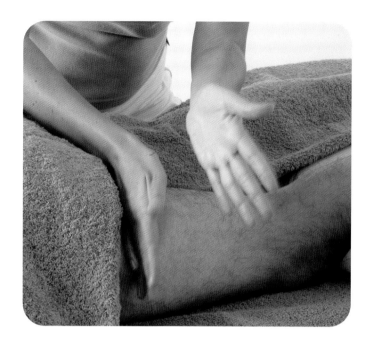

WHAT ARE ITS THERAPEUTIC EFFECTS?

- It draws blood to the skin stimulating the local as well as the overall circulation very effectively.
- Tapotement is invigorating and stimulating.
- Percussion movements cause muscle tissue to contract and therefore induce muscle tone.
- It is often employed over areas such as the thighs or the buttocks to help to break down fatty deposits.

- If performed lightly over the upper back, tapotement can loosen mucous in the lungs and facilitate expectoration. Care should be taken to avoid the spine.
- Gentle percussion may be applied to the abdomen to improve digestion and to help alleviate constipation.

HOW TO DO IT

There are a variety of ways in which tapotement may be performed.

CUPPING is also known as clapping and it is the most common form of percussion. It is performed with the palms of the hands facing downwards and formed into a cup-shape. Alternate hands are then applied to the body in quick succession. The shallow cup shape causes a pocket of air to be trapped against the skin as the hands strike the tissues and a hollow sound is produced. It is easy to tell if it is being produced correctly by listening to the sound. If the hands are kept flat instead of cupped an unpleasant slapping sound may be heard and a stinging sensation is felt!

HACKING is applied with the edge of the hands – the little finger side (the ulnar border of the hands). The wrists need to be very loose so shake your hands out well to relax them. Hold your hands over the body with the palms of your hands facing each other, thumbs uppermost and flick your hands up and down very quickly and rhythmically in rapid succession. The fingers should be loosely held as should the wrists to prevent a heavy karate chopping action!

FLICKING is also known as 'finger-hacking'. It is similar to hacking except that the edges of the little fingers rather than the edges of the hands are bought down into contact with the body. This gives a much lighter effect. The superficial tissues rather than the deep muscles are stimulated.

BEATING AND POUNDING have been grouped together since they are both performed with lightly closed fists. Since beating and pounding are very vigorous they should only be used on the buttocks and fleshy thigh regions. The movements are sometimes referred to as pummelling or both are grouped together as beating. Make your hands into loose fists, and with both hands and wrists relaxed, the fists are applied to the body in quick succession. The movements are light, bouncy and springy rather than heavy and thumping. In pounding, the palmar aspect of the fist is used. In beating the sides of the closed fists are used. These movements are a must for those cellulite thighs!

TAPPING is a very gentle form of tapotement – the French *tapoter* means 'to pat', or 'to drum' (on the table). In contrast to the other percussion movements, this is a very gentle technique. It uses just the fingertips and it is carried out on sensitive, delicate areas such as the face. To perform tapping make sure that the fingers are loose and relaxed and gently tap the fingertips on the area to be treated. The rhythm can be varied – try slow tapping as well as rapid tapping.

LETS PRACTICE!

1. CUPPING (CLAPPING)

A. THE BACK OF THE THIGH

POSITION

At the side of the thigh to be treated.

1. Form a hollow curve with both hands and hold them, palms facing downwards, just above the thigh.

2. Bring your cupped hands down onto the leg in quick succession. Keep your movements light and bouncy. Listen for a hollow sound – if you hear a slapping noise you need to cup your hands more.

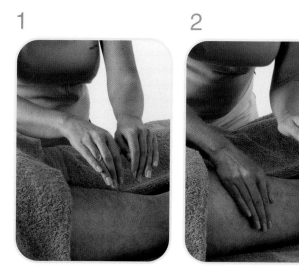

B. THE UPPER BACK

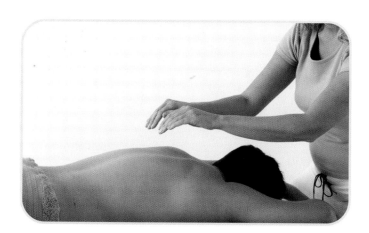

1. Form your hands into a hollow cup shape and hold them palms facing downwards just above the back, one hand either side of the spine. Remember that cupping is never performed over bony prominences.

POSITION

At the head of the receiver.

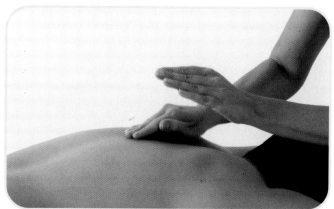

2. Keeping your wrists loose, bring alternate hands down onto the body quickly and rhythmically. Listen for the sound.

Clapping over the upper back is marvellous for relieving congestion from the lungs.

2. HACKING THE OUTER EDGE OF THE THIGH

POSITION

On the opposite side of the thigh to be treated.

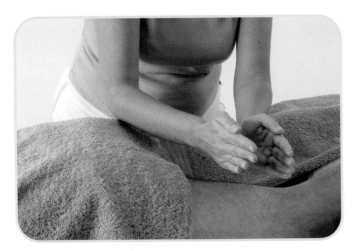

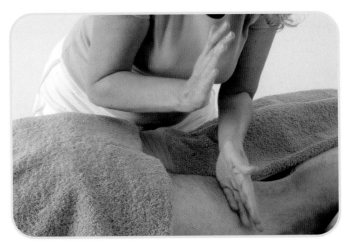

1. Shake your hands out to loosen the wrists and hold your hands over the outer aspect of the thigh with the palms facing each other, thumbs uppermost.

2. Flick them rapidly up and down onto the thigh in quick succession using the sides of your hands. Keep your movements bouncy, light and rhythmical.

3. FLICKING THE UPPER BACK

POSITION

At the side of the receiver facing the upper back.

Place your hands, palms facing each other, thumbs uppermost over the upper back Using the edge of the little fingers only - hence the name 'finger hacking' - let your hands come down on the upper back in a series of rapid light strikes. This produces a much softer effect than the hacking. Do make sure that you do not flick directly onto the spine.

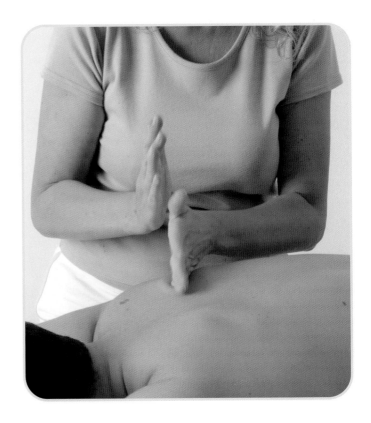

4. BEATING AND POUNDING THE BACK OF THE THIGH

POSITION

On the opposite side of the leg to be treated.

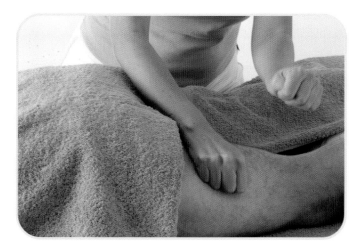

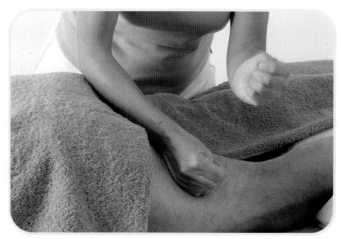

1. Make your hands into loose fists and with hands and wrists relaxed bring the palmar aspects of the fist in contact with the thigh to produce pounding.

2. Still with your fists loosely clenched, this time bounce the sides of your fists alternately against the thigh. This is beating.

5. TAPPING THE FACE

POSITION

At the head of the receiver.

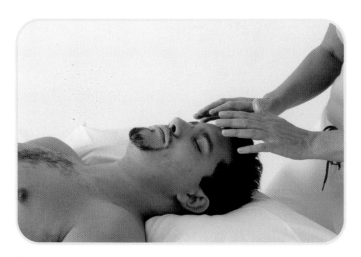

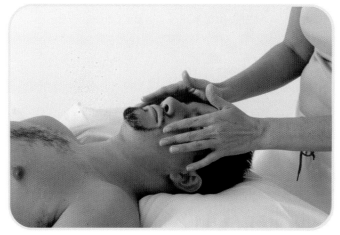

1. Shake out your hands and hold your fingers loosely above the receiver's forehead.

2. Using just the pads of your fingertips, tap very lightly across the forehead, the cheeks and the chin. Try varying the rhythm and notice how tapping can be either soothing or more energising.

VIBRATION

The French word *vibrer* means to vibrate. Vibration is a trembling movement which is performed with one or both hands. It uses either the whole palmar surfaces of the hands or the fingertips. If it performed more vigorously, then it is referred to as 'shaking'. Vibration and shaking are usually classed together. Gentle vibrations and shaking are often given where stronger movements would be uncomfortable.

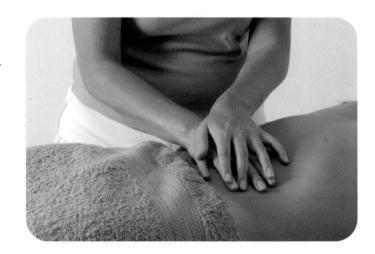

WHAT ARE ITS THERAPEUTIC EFFECTS?

- It may be soothing or stimulating depending on how it is performed.
- Vibration can be used to release pain and tension where muscles are extremely tight and are not responding to other movements.
- It relieves flatulence, indigestion and constipation.

- Vibration stimulates the nerves, together with the muscles supplied by them. This improves their nutrition and helps to restore or maintain their function. Vibration is often used where there is a loss of nerve power as in paralysis.
- Where there are respiration problems, vibration helps to loosen mucous and helps expectoration.

HOW TO DO IT

The palmar surface of one hand or both hands, one on top of the other, are placed on the part to be treated and then the area is vibrated rapidly. Contact is maintained with the area throughout the vibration, and movement may be from side to side or up and down.

Vibration may also be performed gently using just the fingertips along the course of a nerve.

LETS PRACTISE!

Prepare the area before practice with some gentle effleurage movements. Use just a small amount of oil to prevent your hands sliding.

VIBRATION – THE ABDOMEN

POSITION

On the right side of the receiver.

1. Place both hands, palms downwards one on top of the other, onto the receiver's abdomen. To prepare the area for vibration circle around the abdomen moving your hands in a clockwise direction.

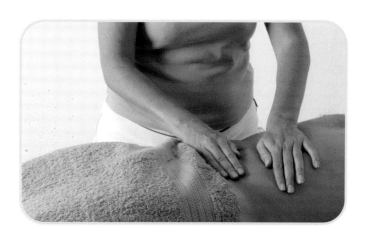

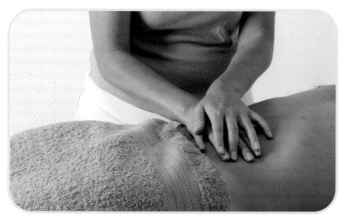

2. Place your hands, one on top of the other on the abdomen and then vibrate your hands rapidly yet gently from side to side.

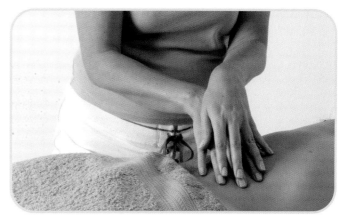

3. Now try the same movement using your fingertips rather than the whole of your hand. Place the fingertips of both hands below the navel and perform gentle vibrations taking care not to prod into the abdomen.

Vibration over the abdomen is excellent for all digestive problems such as constipation and lack of tone.

CHAPTER 3

STEP-BY-STEP MASSAGE

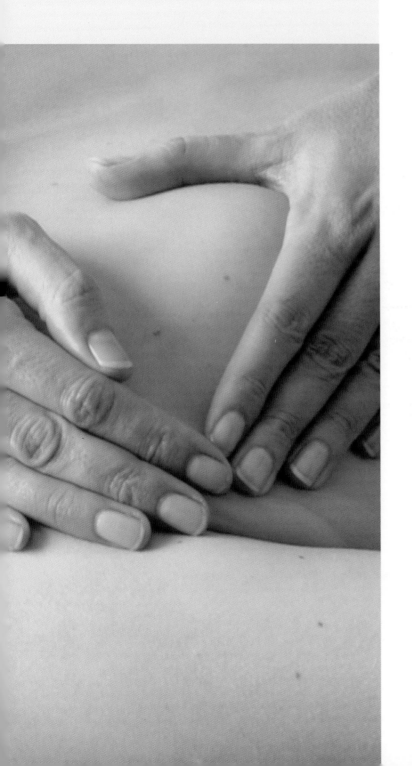

STEP-BY-STEP MASSAGE

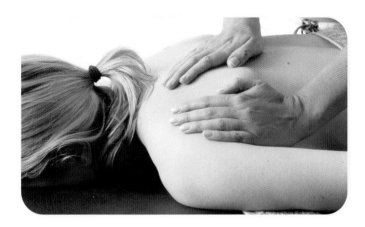

The techniques you have practised in the previous chapter have provided the foundation skills necessary to massage any part of the body. If you decide to carry out a complete body massage you need to allow at least an hour. However, if your time is limited then just concentrate on one or two areas rather than rushing through a full-body massage. It is far better to be thorough! Ask your partner how he or she wishes to feel at the end of the massage. If he or she wants to feel deeply relaxed and even go to sleep, then use lots of effleurage and slow movements to soothe and relax them, omitting the tapotement movements such as cupping and hacking. On the other hand, if he or she wants to feel invigorated and energised, then perform a firmer, brisker massage. My massage sequence is not set in stone for there is no correct sequence for giving a massage.

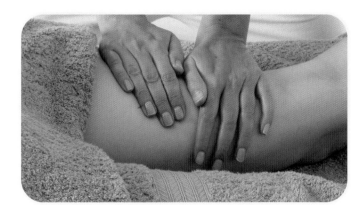

BEFORE YOU BEGIN OBSERVE THE FOLLOWING CHECKLIST:

- Create a warm and relaxing ambience.
- Remove all jewellery from both yourself as well as the receiver.
- Trim your fingernails and make sure that they are clean.
- Wash your hands and if they are cold, warm them.
- Have plenty of cushions, pillows and towels at your disposal to ensure the comfort of both you and the receiver.
- Prepare your massage oil.
- Check for any contraindications.
- Make sure that you are totally relaxed.
- Have a jug of water on hand for use at the end of the massage.

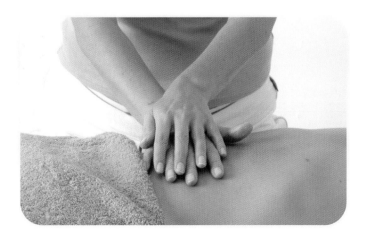

THE BACK

THE BACK IS THE LARGEST AREA YOU
WILL BE MASSAGING AND YOU WILL
SPEND MORE TIME WORKING ON THE
BACK THAN ANY OTHER SINGLE
PART OF THE BODY.

The majority of us will suffer from backache at some time in our
lives and you will be amazed what a difference a back
massage can make. It relaxes tense and knotted muscles
allowing us to release both our physical, as well as emotional
stresses and strains.The receiver should be on his or her front
with one pillow or cushion under the neck and shoulders
(unless you are working on a massage couch with a face hole
ring) and one under their feet. Cover them up completely
with towels.

1. TUNE IN

PURPOSE

■ To establish your initial touch and to induce relaxation.

Allow your hands to rest gently on the receiver's back. Take a
few deep breaths and focus completely on your massage
partner. As you begin to breathe deeply so will the receiver and
any tension will be gently released. Leave your hands there for
about a minute.

POSITION

At the side of the receiver.

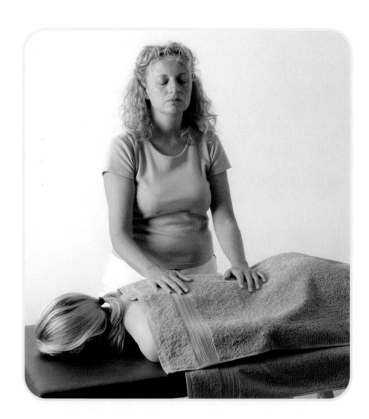

2. OILING

PURPOSE

■ Spreads the massage medium.

POSITION

At the side of the receiver.

1. Draw back the towel. Dispense a small amount of warmed oil into one hand and rub your palms briskly together. Allow your hands to float down onto the back.

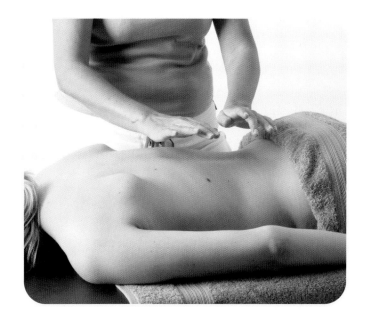

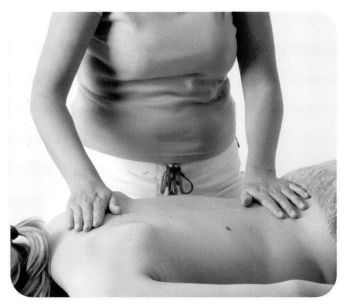

2. With relaxed hands spread the oil slowly all over the back moulding your hands to the contours of the body.

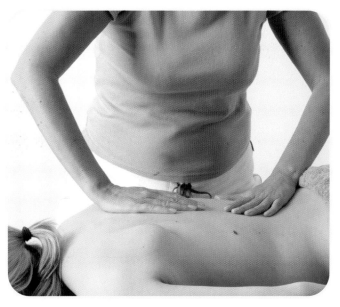

3. Now that you have made contact try not to break it until you have completely finished the back massage.

3. LONG STROKING

A. BOTH HANDS

POSITION

At the side of the receiver.

PURPOSE

- Accustoms the receiver to your touch.
- Deeply relaxes the receiver and warms up the tissues.

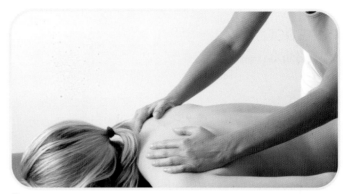

2. Stroke up the entire length of the back and across the shoulders. Maintain a firm pressure and use your body weight.

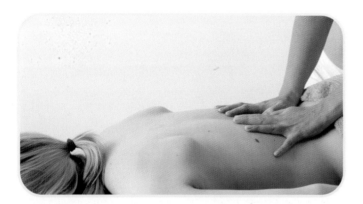

1. Place both hands, flat down, one either side of the spine, at the bottom of the back. Your fingers should face upwards.

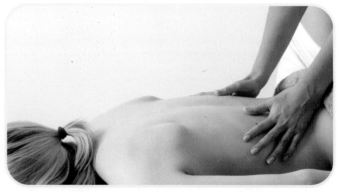

3. Allow your hands to glide back to their starting point lightly skimming across the skin using no pressure whatsoever.

B. ALTERNATE HANDS

PURPOSE

- Accustoms the receiver to your touch.
- Deeply relaxes the receiver and warms up the tissues.

Place both hands, palms downwards, on the lower back. Effleurage firmly up the back and over the shoulder with one hand only and allow it to glide back with no pressure. As the first hand completes the movement repeat the movement with your other hand on the other side of the back. Maintain a smooth and even rhythm as you repeat these movements many times, experimenting with different speeds and pressures.

POSITION

At the side of the receiver.

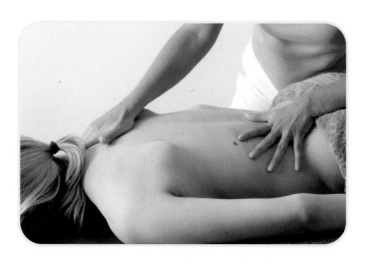

4. CIRCULAR STROKING

POSITION
At the side of the receiver.

PURPOSE
- Deeply relaxes the receiver.
- Warms up the tissues.

1. Place the palms of both hands on the opposite side of the body around the shoulder blade.

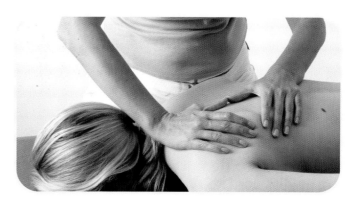

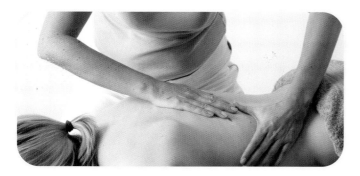

2. Make large stroking movements around the shoulder blade in a circular motion with one hand following the other. As you perform the circles your hands will cross over. Even though you will have to lift one hand over the other, make sure that one hand always has contact with the body.

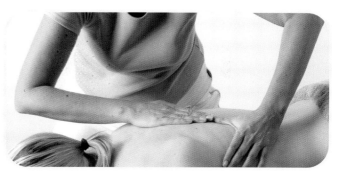

3. Repeat the circular stroking down the body towards the buttock area. Then work back up the body towards the neck.

5. DOUBLE-HANDED CIRCULAR STROKING

PURPOSE
- Deeply relaxes the receiver.
- Warms up the tissues.
- Loosens the muscle fibres.

Put one hand flat on top of the other and place your hands on the opposite side of the body. Make large outward circular movements around the scapula. Continue the reinforced stroking working down towards the buttocks and then back up again. By putting one hand on top of the other with the same effort you will find you can achieve a much deeper pressure.

POSITION
At the side of the receiver.

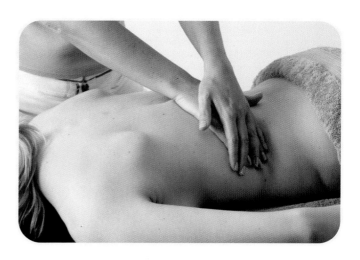

6. FRICTION

POSITION

At the side of the receiver directly over the part to be treated.

PURPOSE

- Enables you to detect any tight areas.
- Breaks up adhesions and nodules.
- Eliminates waste products.
- Brings increased blood flow to the area.

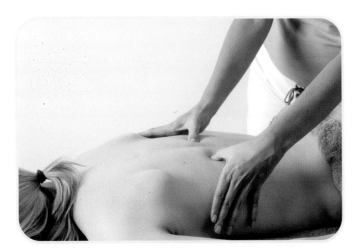

1. Place both hands either side of the spine and put the pads of your thumbs in the dimples at the base of the spine. Perform small, deep circular friction movements gradually working from the dimples up towards the base of the neck.

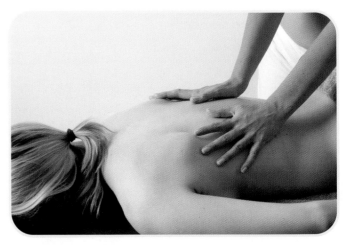

2. As your thumbs are unaccustomed to performing friction they may ache to begin with but they will soon adapt. To increase the pressure and reach the deeper tissues use your body weight to lean into the movement. You may also try stiffening the elbows to achieve more pressure.

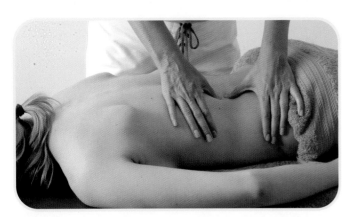

3. If you find a nodule, friction over the area with the ball of your thumb. Friction can be uncomfortable but most people describe it as a 'useful pain'. It should not, however, be too forceful and friction may only be applied for a short period at a time – approximately a minute. You may return to the same area later on in the massage session, but try not to overdo it or the tissues can become irritated.

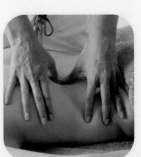

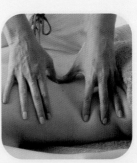

For deeper pressure, place one thumb on top of the other with the fingers splayed out to give support and control, and move your thumbs in a circular direction.

The knuckles may also be used to treat an area with deep friction. Make a fist and place it onto a knotty area and circle over it slowly and deeply.

7. STROKING DOWN THE SIDES OF THE BACK

POSITION

At the side of the receiver.

PURPOSE

■ Flushes away any toxins released.

■ Relieves tension from the muscles.

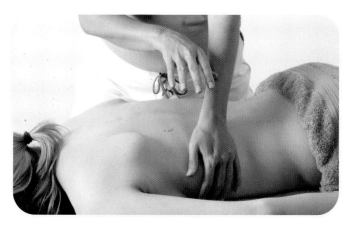

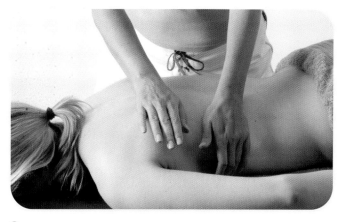

1. Place both hands palms down on the opposite side of the back. Make sure that they are not touching the spine.

2. Using alternate hands, push down first with one hand and then the other, working up and down the back rhythmically.

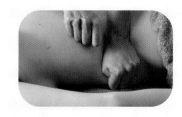

The same movement may be performed with the palmar surface of loosely clenched fists.

8. STROKING THE BUTTOCKS

POSITION

At the side of the receiver, level with the buttocks.

PURPOSE

■ Warms up the area.

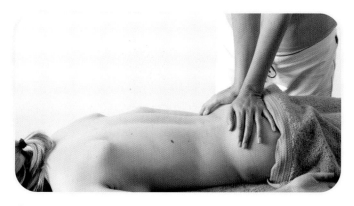

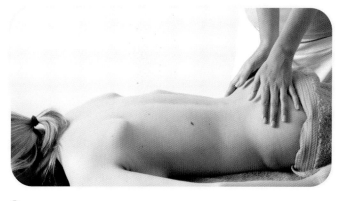

1. Place both hands, palms down, fingers facing upwards, at the top of the buttocks.

2. Stroke up and out across the buttocks. Allow your hands to glide back to your starting position and repeat several times.

9. CIRCULAR STROKING OF THE BUTTOCKS

POSITION

At the side of the receiver, level with the buttocks.

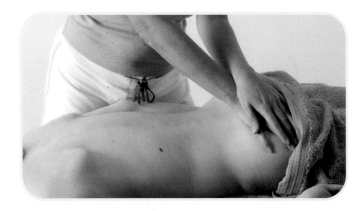

Place one hand flat on top of the other on the opposite buttock. Circle over one buttock and then over the other to produce a large figure-of-eight movement.

PURPOSE

■ Warms up the buttocks.

As a variation, place the palms of both hands around the opposite buttock and make large stroking movements around the buttock making a circle with one hand following the other. Repeat on the other buttock.

10. WRINGING THE BUTTOCKS

POSITION

At the side of the receiver, level with the buttocks.

PURPOSE

■ Improves blood flow and decongests the buttocks.
■ Relieves muscle spasm.
■ Breaks down fatty deposits.
■ Helps to tone the buttocks.

Place both hands, flat down, on the buttocks and with alternate hands rhythmically pick up and wring out the muscles. Ensure that you are picking up as much muscle as possible.

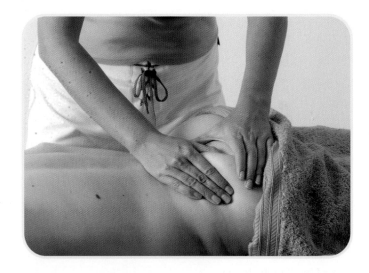

11. PLUCKING THE BUTTOCKS

POSITION

At the side of the receiver, level with the buttocks.

PURPOSE

- Stimulates and tones the buttocks.
- Improves circulation.
- Breaks down fatty deposits.

Use alternate hands to pick up small areas of flesh between your thumbs and fingers. Try to build up a fairly rapid rhythm and make sure that your wrists are loose.

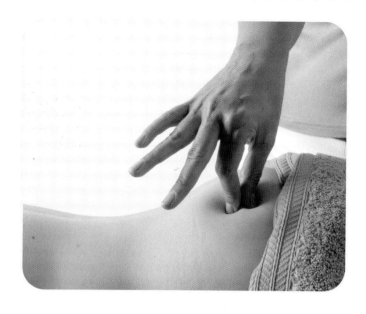

12. FRICTIONING ALONG THE TOP OF THE PELVIS

POSITION

At the side of the receiver, level with the top of the pelvis.

PURPOSE

- Breaks up nodules.
- Disperses toxins.
- Loosens up the pelvis.
- Improves blood flow.

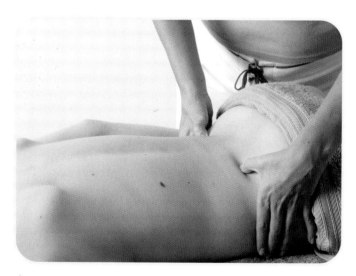

1. Try to locate two dimples at the base of the spine. Use the pads of the thumbs to make small deep circular movements across the pelvis.

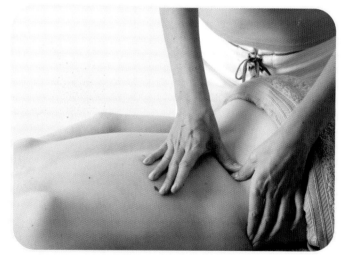

2. If you find a nodule, friction over the area with the ball of one thumb, or place one thumb on top of the other for a deeper pressure. Alternatively, make one hand into a loose fist and circle it slowly and deeply over a knotty area.

13. PERCUSSION OF THE BUTTOCKS

POSITION

At the side of the receiver, level with the buttocks.

PURPOSE

■ Induces muscle tone.

■ Invigorates and stimulates.

■ Breaks down fatty deposits and congestion.

1. Form your hands into a hollow curve and hold them over the buttock area, palms facing downwards in preparation for cupping. Keeping your wrists loose, bring alternate hands onto the body rapidly and rhythmically. Hold your hands over the buttocks with the palms facing each other, thumbs uppermost. Flick them up and down briskly in quick succession, using the sides of your hands.

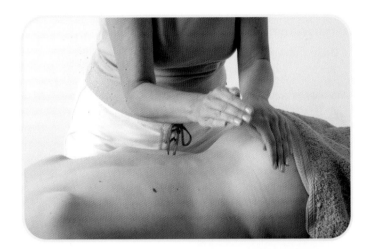

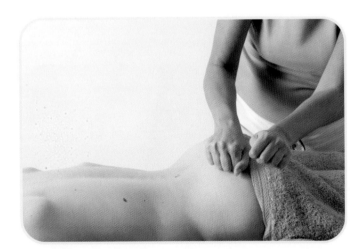

2. Make your hands into loose fists and bring the palmar aspects of both hands down onto the buttocks to produce pounding.

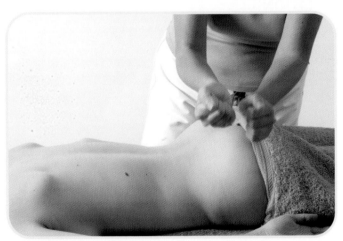

3. To perform beating, bounce the sides of your fists alternately against the buttocks.

14. CIRCLE STROKING OF THE SHOULDER BLADES

POSITION

At the side of the receiver, level with the shoulder blades.

PURPOSE

- Warms up the area.
- Loosens tension.
- Prepares the shoulder blades for deeper work.

1. As we have treated the lower back, cover up this area by bringing the towel halfway up the back to keep it warm. Place the palms of both hands on the opposite side of the body around the shoulder blade.

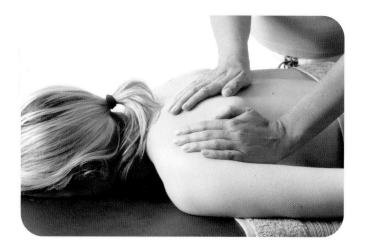

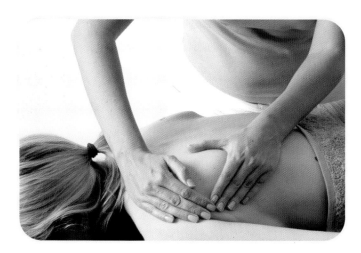

2. Make large stroking movements around the shoulder blade in a circular motion, with one hand following the other. As you perform the circles, your hands will cross over. Even though you will have to lift one hand over the other, make sure that one hand always has contact with the body.

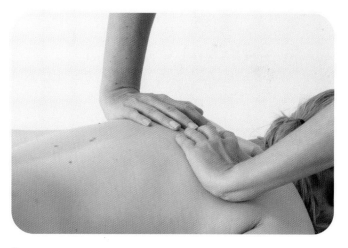

3. Place one palm on the right shoulder blade and one on the left, and make large outward circles, using both hands simultaneously. As a variation, position yourself at the receiver's head. Carry out the procedure from this position.

15. SQUEEZING THE SHOULDER BLADE

POSITION

At the side of the receiver level with the shoulder blade to be treated.

1. Place the receiver's arm gently behind their back. With one hand support the shoulder from underneath and place your other hand around the bottom of the scapula with the thumb and forefinger spread out so that your hand fits the shape of the shoulder blade. Gently squeeze the shoulder blade with your upper hand.

2. Use your thumb and fingers to gently squeeze the upper part of the scapula.

PURPOSE

- Releases toxins.
- Loosens the scapula.
- Relieves muscle spasm.
- Brings an increased blood supply to the area.

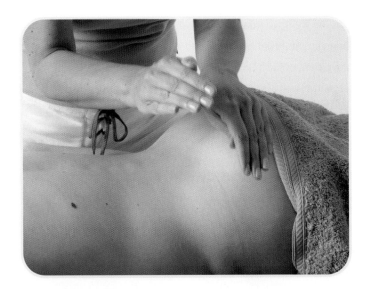

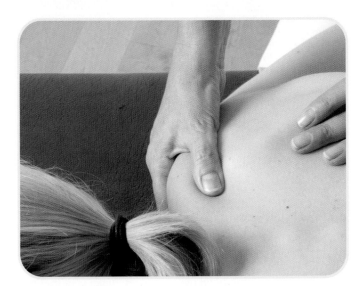

16. FRICTIONING THE SHOULDER BLADE

POSITION

At the side of the receiver.

PURPOSE

- Releases knots and nodules.
- Improves mobility.
- Eliminates waste products.
- Increases blood flow.
- Gives pain relief.

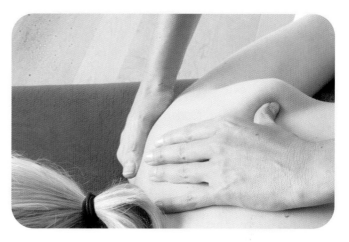

1. Place one hand under the shoulder for support and use the thumb of your other hand to apply deep, circular, friction movements all around the rim of the shoulder blade.

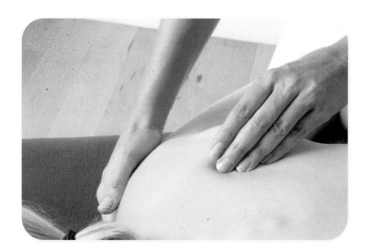

2. You may also use your fingertips to friction around the shoulder blade. You will find many knots and nodules which you should try to break down using the balls of the thumbs or by gentle knuckling.

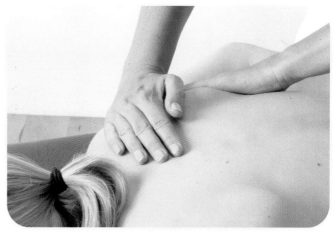

3. After completing the friction movements, perform circular effleurage around the area working towards the axilla (armpit) to drain away any toxins that have been released.

17. WRINGING THE SHOULDERS

POSITION

At the side of the receiver level with the neck and shoulders.

PURPOSE

- Brings a fresh blood supply to the area.
- Loosens the shoulders.
- Decongests the area.
- Relieves muscle spasm.

Using alternate hands, rhythmically pick up and wring the top of the shoulders, gathering up the maximum amount of flesh.

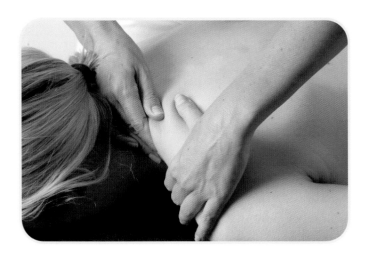

18. PICKING UP AND SQUEEZING THE NECK

POSITION

At the side of the receiver facing the neck.

PURPOSE

- Loosens the neck.
- Eliminates toxins.
- Relieves and prevents muscle stiffness.

If you are working on a couch, the receiver can use the face hole. Otherwise, the receiver should rest his or her forehead on their hands to straighten out the neck – a small rolled up towel or pillow under the head is optional. Place both hands, flat down, on the back of the neck and gently pick up and squeeze the muscles at the back of the neck.

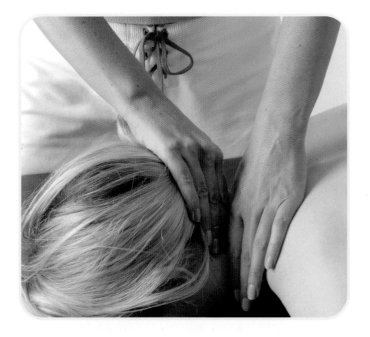

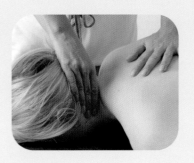

This technique may be performed using both hands at once or one hand may follow the other.

19. STROKING THE BACK

POSITION

Above the receiver's head.

1. Place both hands, palms down and fingers pointing downwards at the top of the shoulders with one hand either side of the spine.

PURPOSE

- Relaxes the receiver.
- Drains away toxins.

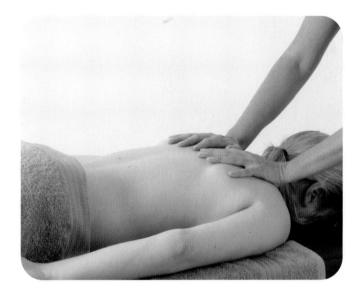

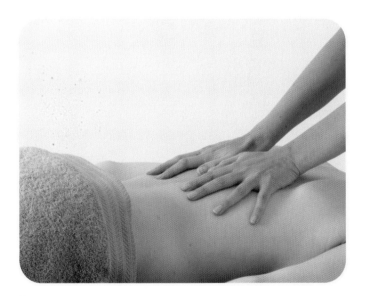

2. Effleurage down the whole length of the back and out across the buttocks. Allow your hands to glide back with no pressure whatsoever.

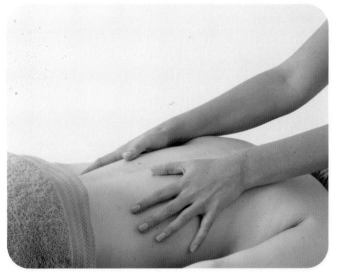

3. As a variation, place your palms on either side of the upper back with the fingers pointing towards the spine. The fingertips should be by the side of, but not directly on top of, the spine. Stroke down the back and across the buttocks. Allow your hands to glide gently back with no pressure.

20. CAT STROKING OF THE BACK

POSITION

At the side of the receiver.

PURPOSE

Completely relaxes the receiver.

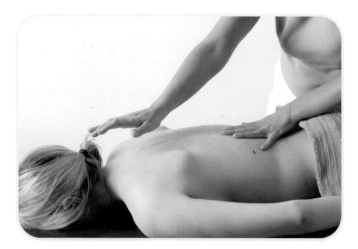

1. Place the whole of the palm of one hand at the base of the receiver's neck. Stroke slowly down the body using very little pressure. As you lift off one hand when it reaches the buttocks, repeat the movement with the other hand. Make sure that, at no time, contact is lost with the receiver. It should feel like one continuous movement.

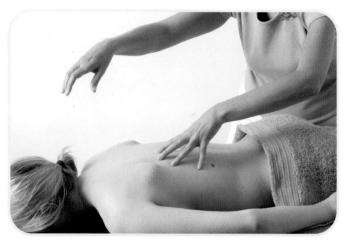

2. As a variation, repeat the same technique using just the fingertips of your hands so that they are barely touching the skin.

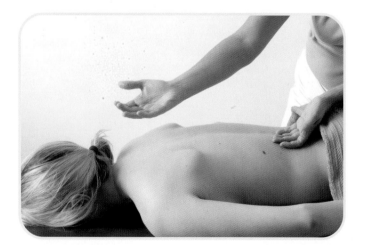

3. Alternatively, carry out the procedure using the backs of your hands.

YOUR BACK MASSAGE IS NOW COMPLETE!

COVER THE BACK WITH A TOWEL AND ALLOW YOUR MASSAGE PARTNER TO RELAX DEEPLY.

THE BACK OF THE LEG

1. OILING

POSITION

At the side of the leg to be massaged.

PURPOSE

- Establishes contact.
- Spreads the massage medium.
- Accustoms the receiver to your touch.

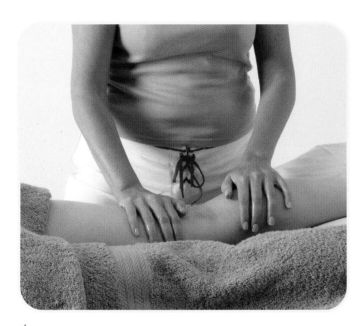

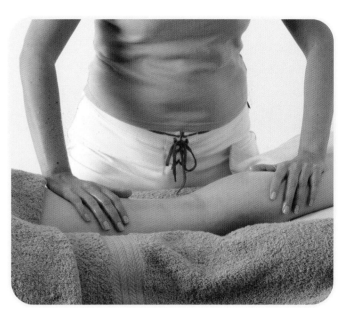

1. Draw back the towel, exposing only one leg – the one you are not treating should be left covered up. Dispense a small amount of warmed oil onto one hand and rub your palms together. Lower your hands gently down onto the leg and simply rest them there for a few minutes to establish initial contact.

2. Spread the oil slowly onto the leg, making sure that it is thoroughly dispersed.

2. STROKING

POSITION
At the side of the receiver.

PURPOSE
- Brings fresh blood to the area.
- Prepares the tissues for deeper movements.
- Helps to flush away toxins.

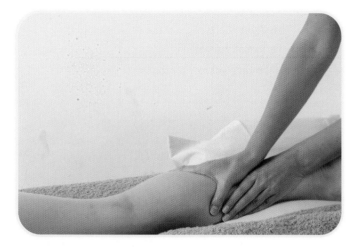

1. Place both hands, palms down, in a V-shape just above the heel. One hand should be just above the other.

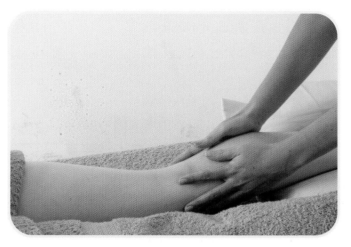

2. Stroke firmly up the calf and thigh muscles, moulding your hands to the contours of the leg. Apply very little pressure to the back of the knee, since it is a delicate area.

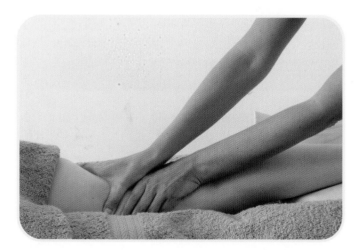

3. As your hands reach the top of the thigh, allow them to separate and glide them back down the sides of the leg using virtually no pressure whatsoever. Repeat these strokes many times, gradually increasing the pressure.

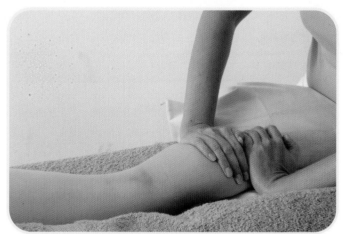

4. As a variation, place one hand across the back of the ankle with the fingertips pointing in one direction and your other hand just above with fingertips pointing in the other direction. Effleurage up the leg, taking care over the back of the knee, fan your hands out at the top of the thigh just as you did previously and allow your hands to glide gently back to your starting point. Repeat this movement many times.

3. DRAINING THE CALF

POSITION

At the side of the calf.

1. Gently lift the foot and lower leg, supporting it comfortably with your hand and forearm.

PURPOSE

■ Encourages drainage of toxins.

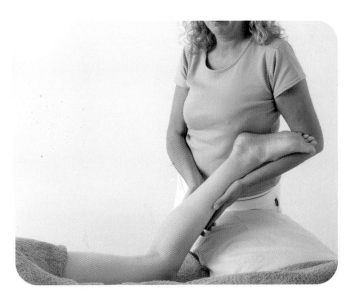

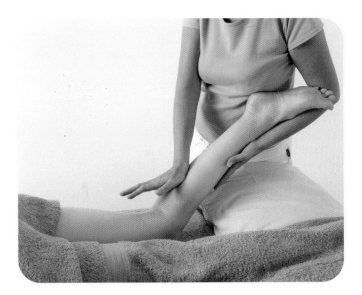

2. Use the heel of your other hand to stroke from the foot to the back of the knee.

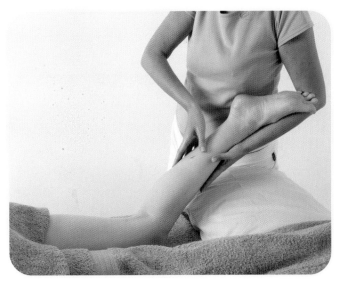

3. Then allow your hand to glide gently back. Repeat this movement several times and then gently lower the leg.

4. PICKING UP, SQUEEZING AND ROLLING THE LEG

POSITION

At the side of the leg.

PURPOSE

- Increases blood supply to the area.
- Decongests.
- Relieves muscle spasm.
- Breaks down fatty deposits.

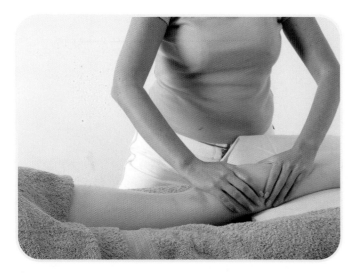

1. Place both hands, palms down, on the calf with your thumbs well outstretched.

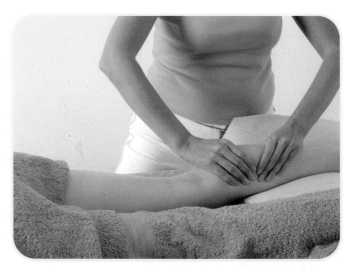

2. Gently and slowly lift the muscle away from the bone and squeeze and release it. Repeat the picking up and squeezing along the entire leg and then back down again.

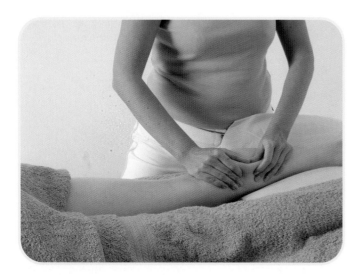

3. Starting at the lower calf with your hands in the same position, pick up the muscle and roll the thumbs towards the fingers. Work all the way up the leg and back down again.

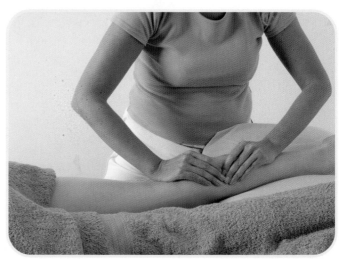

4. Repeat the rolling action but this time roll your fingers towards the thumbs.

5. WRINGING THE LEG

POSITION

At the side of the leg. Wringing can be performed from the same or the opposite side.

PURPOSE

- Aids the removal of toxins from the deeper tissues.
- Delivers fresh blood to the leg.
- Relieves stiffness.
- Softens fatty deposits and eliminates.

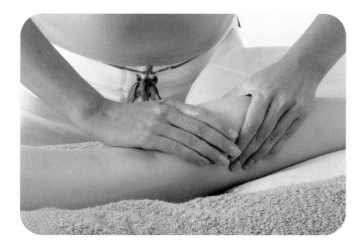

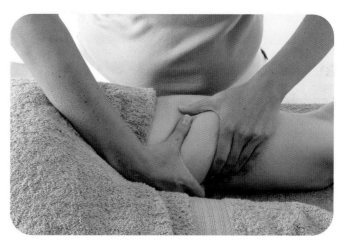

1. Use alternate hands to pick up and wring the leg muscles with a motion similar to wringing out a chamois leather.

2. Make your movements smooth and rhythmic without pinching as you work all the way up to the top of the leg and back down again.

6. CRISS-CROSSING THE LEG

POSITION

At the side of the leg.

PURPOSE

- Eliminates the toxins.
- Improves circulation.
- Alleviates muscular tightness.

Place your hands, palms down, on either side of the leg with your fingertips facing away from you. Pull one hand towards you whilst you push away and down with the other hand. Maintain a steady and even rhythm as you criss-cross the entire leg, as usual taking care at the back of the knee.

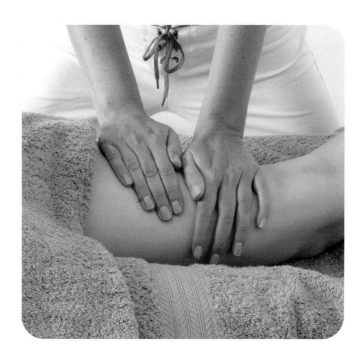

7. PERCUSSION OF THE LEG

POSITION

At the side of the leg.

PURPOSE

- Improves muscle tone in the legs.
- Reduces fatty deposits and cellulite.
- Stimulates the circulation.
- Enlivens the whole body.

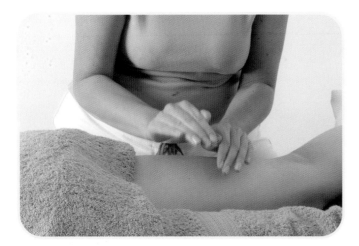

1. Form a hollow curve with both hands and hold them, palms facing downwards, just above the thigh.

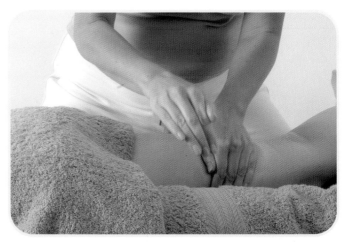

2. Bring your cupped hands down onto the leg in quick succession. Keep your movements light and bouncy. Listen for a hollow sound – if you hear a slapping noise you need to cup your hands more. Repeat the cupping along the entire leg, avoiding the back of the knee.

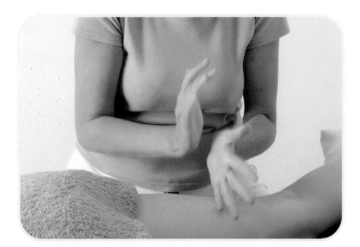

3. Shake your hands out to loosen the wrists and hold your hands over the leg with the palms facing each other, thumbs uppermost. Flick them rapidly up and down onto the thigh in quick succession using the side of your hands. Keep your movements bouncy, light and rhythmical.

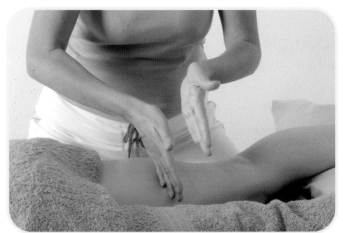

4. Place your hands, palms facing each other, thumbs uppermost, over the leg. Using the edge of the little fingers only – hence the name 'finger-hacking' – let your hands come down on the upper back in a series of rapid light strikes. This produces a much softer effect than the hacking.

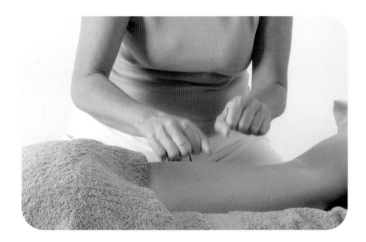

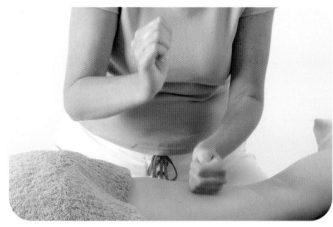

5. Make your hands into loose fists and with hands and wrists relaxed, bring the palmar aspects of the fist in contact with the thigh to produce pounding.

6. Keep your fists loosely clenched, but this time bounce the sides of your fists alternately against the leg. This is beating.

8. FINGERTIP STROKING

POSITION
At the foot of the receiver.

PURPOSE
■ Induces a deep sense of relaxation.

Place the fingertips of one hand at the top of the thigh and stroke gently down with a feather-light touch. As one hand reaches the foot, lift it off gently and use the other hand to start again at the top of the thigh. It should feel like one continuous stroke to the receiver. Stroke more and more gently continuing for as long as you like.

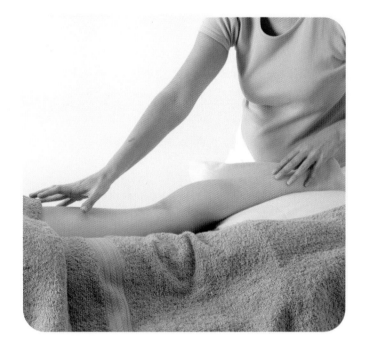

YOU HAVE NOW COMPLETED THE BACK OF THE LEG.
REPEAT ON THE OTHER LEG AND THEN COVER BOTH LEGS WITH A TOWEL.

THE UPPER CHEST, NECK AND HEAD

Ask the receiver to turn over onto his or her back so that you can massage the front of the body. Remember to place a pillow or cushion under the head, one under the knees to take the strain off the lower back and any other cushions you wish to use to ensure the comfort of you and your partner.

1. OILING

POSITION

At the head of the receiver.

PURPOSE

- Re-establishes contact now that the receiver has turned over.
- Spreads the massage oil.

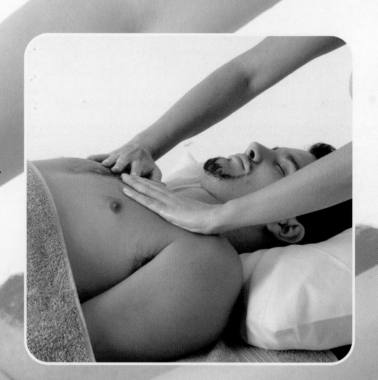

Dispense a small amount of oil onto the palm of one hand and rub your hands together to warm it slightly. Lower your hands gently down onto the chest holding them just below the collar bones, fingers pointing towards one another. Encourage the receiver to breathe deeply and as they fall into a deep state of relaxation begin to spread the oil by stroking the whole area.

2. STROKING THE CHEST

POSITION

At the head of the receiver.

1. With your hands placed just below the collarbone, fingertips pointing towards each other, effleurage out across the chest.

PURPOSE

- Warms up the chest.
- Prepares the chest for deeper movements.
- Encourages the elimination of toxins.

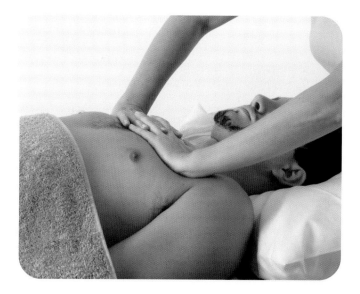

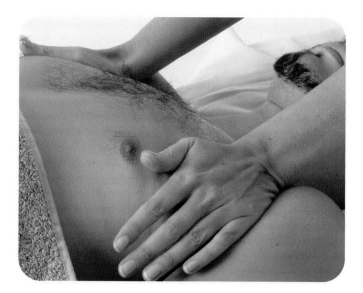

2. Then slide your hands down towards the armpits to encourage drainage.

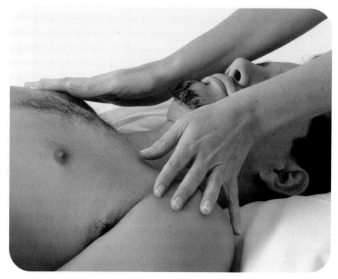

3. Glide your hands gently back to your starting point using no pressure whatsoever. Repeat several times.

3. MASSAGING THE CLAVICLES (COLLARBONE)

POSITION

At the head of the receiver.

PURPOSE

- Loosens the chest.
- Releases the chest muscles.
- Relieves congestion from the chest.
- Brings fresh blood to the area.

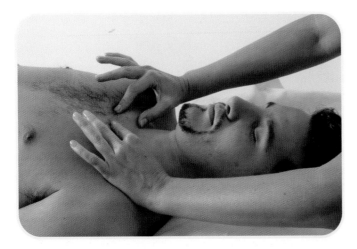

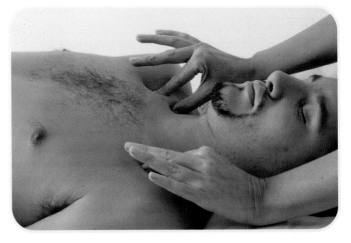

1. Place the thumbs on one side of the collarbone and your forefingers on the other and run them gently along the collarbone, working from the centre of the chest outwards.

2. Using the thumbs and forefinger, very gently squeeze and release the collarbone.

4. FRICTIONING THE CLAVICLES (COLLARBONE)

POSITION

At the head of the receiver.

PURPOSE

- Breaks up nodules.
- Loosens up the shoulder girdle.
- Increases blood flow to the area.
- Dispels accumulated waste products.

Place the pads of the thumbs towards the centre of the chest just below the clavicles. Perform small circular friction movements, working along the collarbone towards the shoulders.

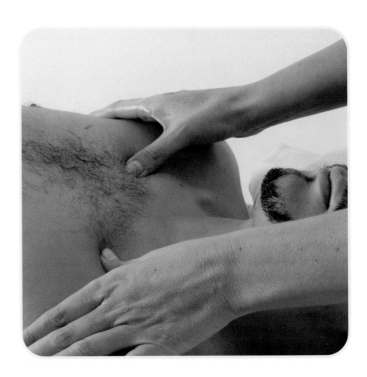

5. KNUCKLING THE CHEST

POSITION

At the head of the receiver.

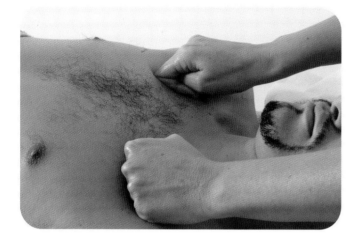

1. Make both hands into loose fists and place them near the middle of the chest just below the collarbone. Slide your knuckles gently outwards across the chest and allow them to glide back again.

PURPOSE

- Breaks down knots and nodules.
- Releases deeper toxins.
- Brings blood to the area.

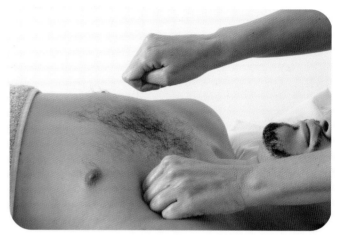

2. Perform small circular movements with your knuckles all over the chest area. You must press lightly on this delicate area.

6. PICKING UP AND SQUEEZING THE CHEST

POSITION

At the head of the receiver.

PURPOSE

- Releases tension in the chest.
- Decongests the area.

Place both hands palms down onto the fleshy area in front of one of the armpits. Gently pick up and squeeze the muscle using alternate hands. Repeat on the other side.

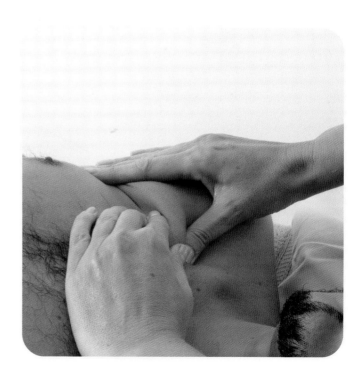

7. TAPPING THE CHEST

POSITION

At the head of the receiver.

PURPOSE

- Breaks down mucous relieving congestion.
- Stimulates the area.
- Tones the muscles.

Make sure that your fingers are loose and relaxed and hold them just above the chest area. Use the pads of the fingertips to tap very lightly all across the chest area.

8. STROKING THE CHEST

POSITION

At the head of the receiver.

PURPOSE

- Completes the chest massage.
- Drains away toxins.
- Relaxes and soothes.

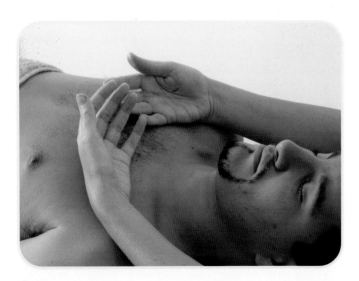

1. To complete the chest massage, place the backs of your hands just below the collarbone with your fingertips pointing towards each other.

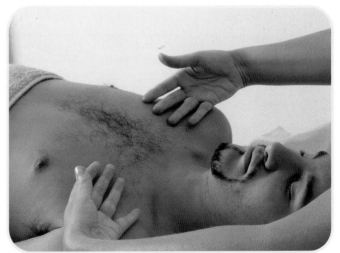

2. Very gently stroke out across the chest and towards the lymph glands under the arms.

9. RELEASING THE NECK

POSITION

At the head of the receiver.

1. Dispense a small amount of oil onto your hands. Bring both hands, palms facing up, under the receiver's neck so that your fingertips are touching.

PURPOSE

■ Dissolves muscular tension in the neck.

■ Relaxes the receiver.

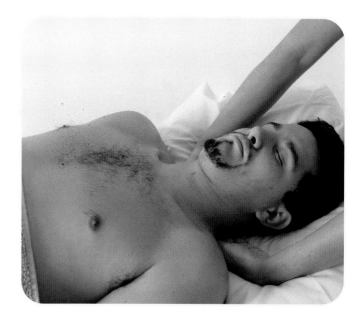

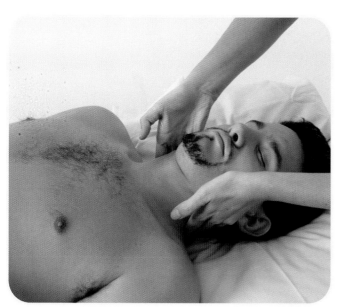

2. Use both hands to gently pull up the muscles of both sides of the neck towards you.

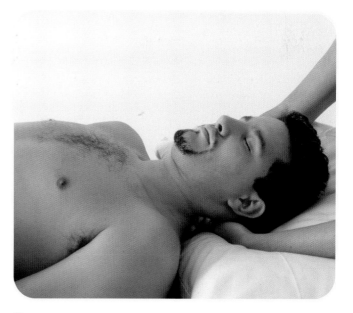

3. As a variation, place both hands under the receiver's neck with one hand above the other, and gently pull both sides of the neck upwards towards you.

10. FRICTIONING THE NECK

POSITION
At the head of the receiver.

PURPOSE
- Releases tense, knotty muscles.
- Prevents headaches.
- Stimulates blood flow.

Place the fleshy pads of your fingers at the base of the receiver's neck on either side of the spine. Perform small, circular movements working up towards the base of the skull. Make sure that you are not pressing on the spine. Continue your circular pressures underneath the bony ridge at the base of the skull using the two middle fingers of each hand.

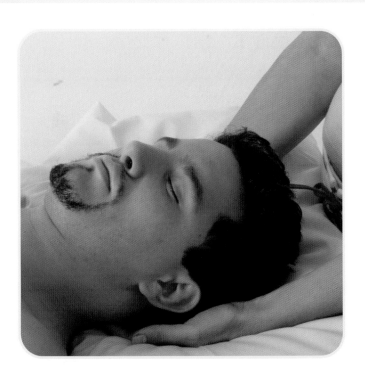

11. STROKING THE NECK

POSITION
At the head of the receiver.

PURPOSE
- Releases neck tension.
- Drains toxins.
- Stretches the neck gently.

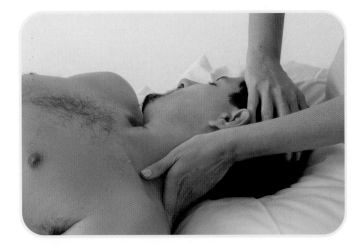

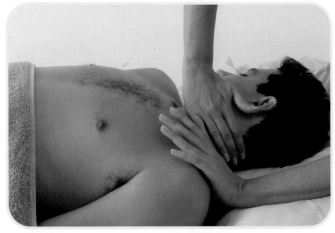

1. Place both hands on the side of the neck and turn the head very gently to the side. It is important never to force the neck. Now place one hand on the back of the head and use the other hand to stroke down the side of the neck from the base of the skull towards the shoulder.

2. As a variation, stroke one hand down the side of the neck and as it reaches the shoulder begin to stroke with your other hand. Repeat these movements on the other side of the neck.

12. FRICTIONING THE SIDE OF THE NECK

POSITION

At the head of the receiver.

PURPOSE

- Breaks down knots.
- Gently stretches the neck.
- Eliminates toxins.
- Releases nervous tension.

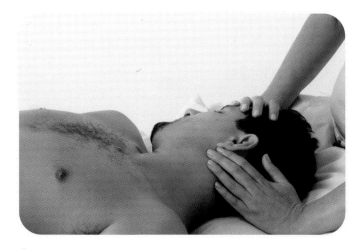

1. With the head still turned to the side, support the receiver's head with one hand and place the fingertips of your other hand on the side of the neck just below the ear.

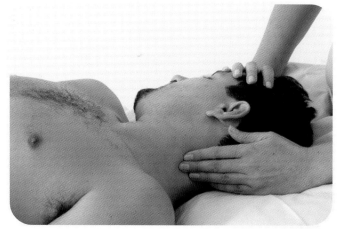

2. Perform slow circles all the way down the side of the neck paying particular attention to any areas of tightness. Use gentle pressure, and always follow friction of the neck with some light stroking as described in the previous step.

13. TUNING IN TO THE FACE

POSITION

At the head of the receiver.

PURPOSE

- Accustoms the receiver to your touch.
- Releases anxiety.

Rest the palms of your hands lightly on the receiver's forehead for a few moments.

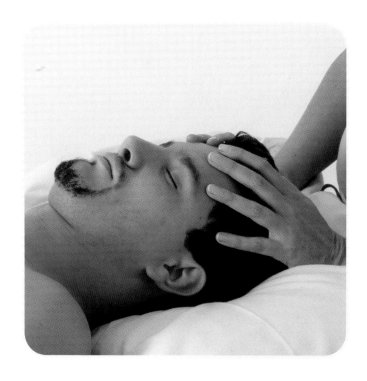

14. STROKING THE FACE

POSITION

At the head of the receiver.

PURPOSE

- Gives a healthy, vibrant glow to the skin.
- Induces peace and serenity.
- Relaxes taut muscles in the face.
- Releases tension.
- Drains away toxins.

1. Dispense a small amount of oil into your hands – take care not to use too much as your massage partner will not want to look oily at the end of the treatment. The oil you use should be absorbed by the skin. Place the palms of your hands on the receiver's forehead with your fingers interlocking and gently stroke outwards across the forehead.

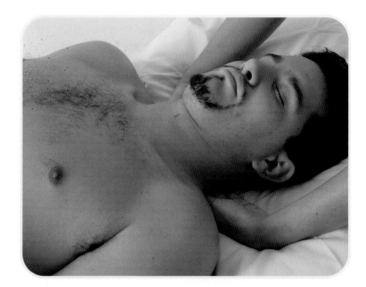

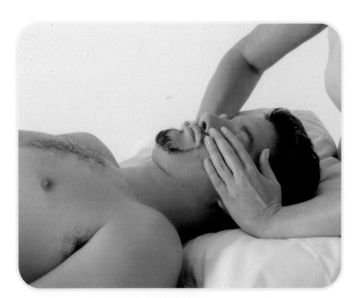

2. Place one hand on each of the receiver's cheeks and stroke with your fingertips out across the cheeks.

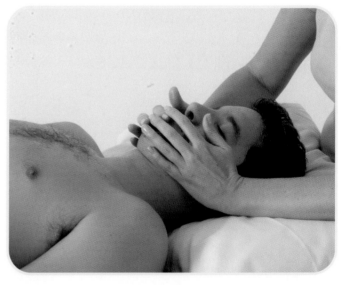

3. Place your fingers in the centre of the receiver's chin and stroke outwards and then continue the movement down the neck and towards the shoulders.

15. PRESSING AND DRAINING THE FOREHEAD

POSITION

At the head of the receiver.

1. Place your thumbs in the centre of the forehead just below the hairline. Imagine that the forehead is divided into horizontal strips about two centimetres (half an inch) wide. Press your thumbs gently and then glide them out across the forehead. Return your thumbs to the forehead and begin the next strip, once again pressing and then draining outwards. Continue down the forehead until you reach the receiver's eyebrows.

PURPOSE

- Improves circulation to the face.
- Releases and drains away impurities.
- Relaxes taut muscles.

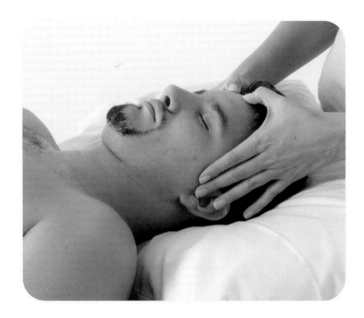

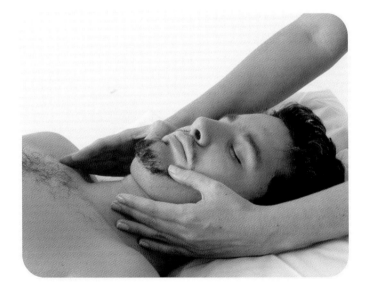

2. Now place your thumbs just under the inner corners of the eyes. Press gently in with the pads of your thumbs and stroke outwards across the cheeks. Work down the entire cheek area in horizontal strips. If you prefer you may use the pad of the forefinger or the middle finger depending upon the size of the face and the size of your fingers.

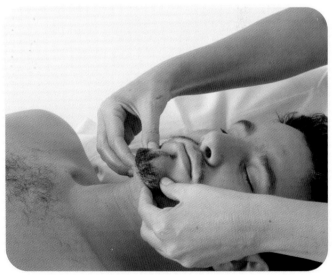

3. Place your thumbs in the centre of the chin just below the mouth and once again press and drain outwards. Treat the whole of the chin in this way. When you have pressed and drained the entire face it is advisable to effleurage the face once more as described in the previous step to drain away any waste products.

16. SMOOTHING AND SQUEEZING THE EYEBROWS

POSITION

At the head of the receiver.

PURPOSE

- Tones the eyebrows.
- Encourages healthier-looking eyebrows.

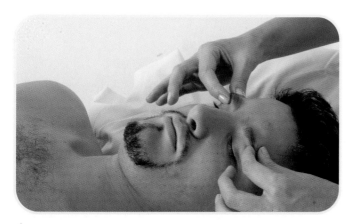

1. Rest your thumbs gently on the inner aspect of the eyebrows and draw your thumbs out to the side along the eyebrows.

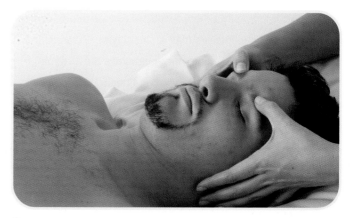

2. Use your thumb and index finger to lightly squeeze the brow bone working from the inner to the outer edges.

17. DRAINING THE NOSE

POSITION

At the head of the receiver.

PURPOSE

- Accustoms the receiver to your touch.

Use the pads of both thumbs, index or middle fingers to stroke down the sides of the nose.

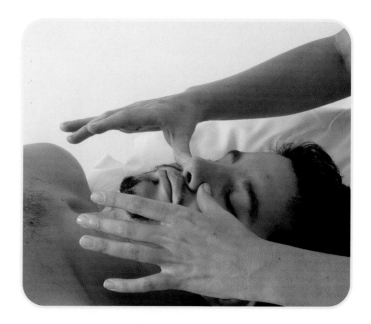

18. MASSAGING THE EARS

POSITION

At the head of the receiver.

PURPOSE

- Induces pleasure.
- Relieves tension.

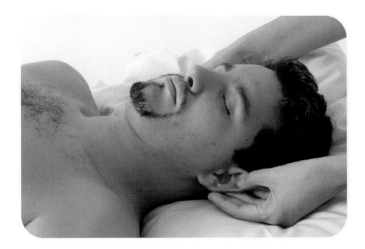

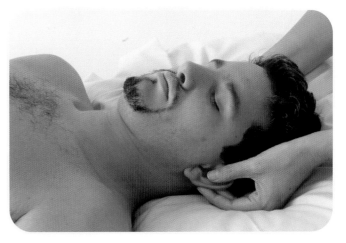

1. Use your thumbs and forefingers to squeeze and massage all over the ears. Then run your fingertips up and down the back of the ears where they connect to the head.

2. Finally, slowly and gently stretch them away from the head.

19. MASSAGING THE JAW LINE

POSITION

At the head of the receiver.

PURPOSE

- Releases tension from the jaw.
- Reduces stress.
- Excellent for teeth grinders.

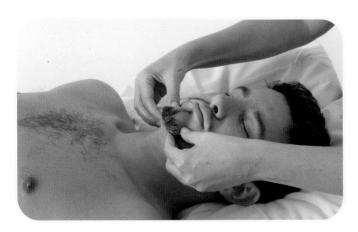

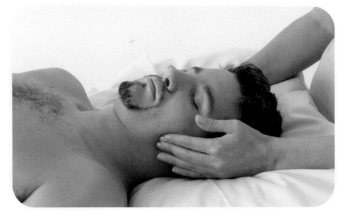

1. Place your hands in the centre of the receiver's jaw, thumbs above the jaw line and fingertips below. Using your thumbs and forefingers gently squeeze and release at regular intervals all along the jaw line.

2. When you have almost reached the ears, perform small circles over the chewing muscles with the pads of your fingertips.

20. DISSOLVING SCALP TENSION

PURPOSE

- Stimulates hair growth.
- Releases tension from the scalp.
- Relieves headaches.
- Improves concentration.

Place the fleshy pads of your fingers and thumbs, well spread out, onto the receiver's scalp. Using fairly firm pressure slowly massage the entire scalp using circular movements.

POSITION

At the head of the receiver.

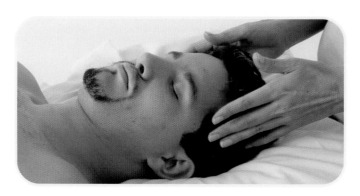

21. TUGGING THE HAIR

PURPOSE

- Releases tightness around the scalp.
- Encourages hair growth.
- Improves the condition of the hair.

Begin by gently combing through the hair using all your fingers. Then gather up small handfuls of hair and gently tug them.

POSITION

At the head of the receiver.

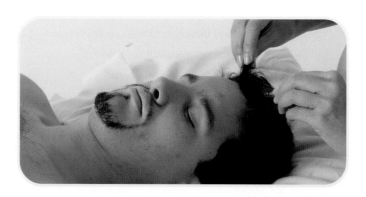

22. TAPPING THE FACE AND SCALP

PURPOSE

- Tones the muscles.
- Energises the face and scalp.

Using just the pads of your fingertips tap very lightly all over the receiver's scalp. Then tap across the forehead, the cheeks and the chin. To finish the head massage, place your hands on either side of the receiver's head.

POSITION

At the head of the receiver.

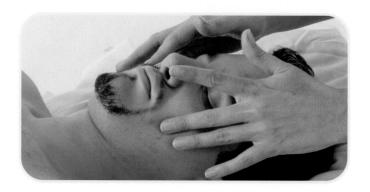

YOU HAVE NOW COMPLETED THE CHEST, NECK AND HEAD MASSAGE.

THE ARM AND HAND

1. OILING

POSITION
At the side of the arm to be treated.

PURPOSE
- Establishes contact with the arm.
- Spreads the massage medium.

Place both hands, palms downwards, across the receiver's wrist and glide them both up the arm.

Uncover one of the arms and arrange it at the side with the palm turned down on the towel.

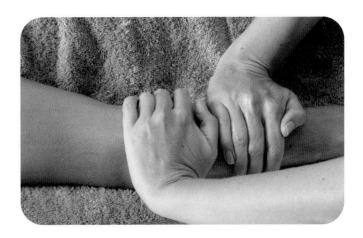

2. STROKING THE ARM

POSITION
At the side of the receiver's arm.

PURPOSE
- Assists the circulation.
- Aids the lymphatic system.
- Prepares the arm for deeper movements.

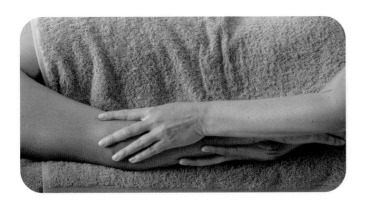

1. Support the forearm underneath with one hand and effleurage up the arm with the other hand.

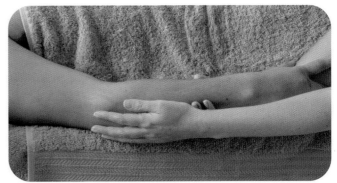

2. Allow the hand to glide back, with no pressure, towards its starting point.

Change hands and repeat the effleurage. This technique ensures that all aspects of the arm are treated. It should feel like one continuous stroke.

3. PETRISSAGE THE UPPER ARM

POSITION

At the side of the receiver's arm.

PURPOSE

- Brings the deeper toxins to the surface.
- Releases muscular tension.
- Stretches the arm.
- Delivers an increased blood supply to the area.
- Breaks down fatty deposits.

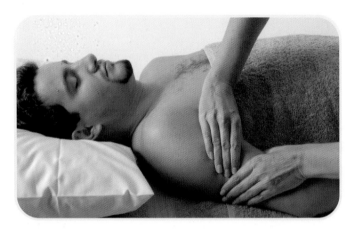

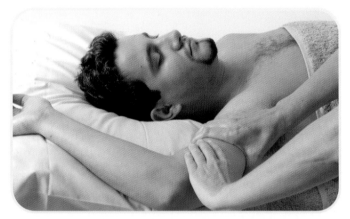

1. Use both hands to rhythmically pick up and squeeze and wring the muscles of the upper arm.

2. To wring the muscles on the other side of the upper arm gently lift the arm with the elbow bent over the head. Do not pinch the flesh.

4. LOOSENING THE ELBOW

POSITION

At the side of the elbow.

The simplest way to work on the elbows is to bend the receiver's elbow and place it across the upper body. This leaves you with both hands free to massage. Use the pads of your fingers and thumb to massage all around the bony surface of the elbow, performing tiny circular pressures over the entire elbow. This tends to be a dry area so you may need a little extra oil. You may also work gently into the crook of the elbow, but do take care since this is a delicate area.

PURPOSE

- Loosens the elbow.
- Increases the circulation.
- Assists the elimination of toxins.

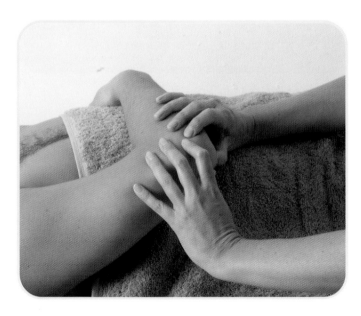

5. DRAINING THE FOREARM

POSITION
At the side of the lower arm.

PURPOSE
- Drains the toxins from the forearm.

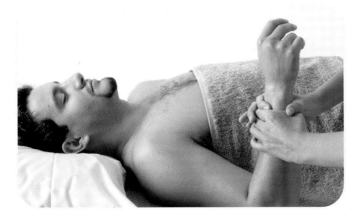

1. Leave the upper arm on the massage surface, but bend the elbow to raise the forearm. Make a ring around the receiver's wrist using the thumbs and fingers of both your hands – your thumbs should be on the inside of the wrist, one above the other.

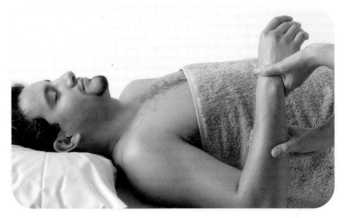

2. Slide both hands slowly and gently down the forearm. As you reach the crook of the arm allow your hands to slide back again with no pressure.

6. LOOSENING THE WRIST

PURPOSE
- Improves mobility in the wrist.
- Breaks down old scar tissue.

POSITION
At the side of the wrist.

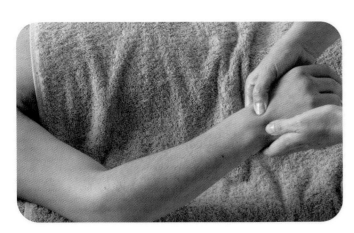

1. Use both thumbs either together or alternately to perform small circular movements both on the outside and the inside of the wrist.

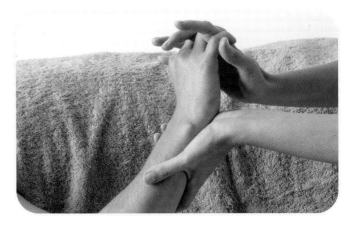

2. Interlock your fingers with the receiver's and move the wrist clockwise and anti-clockwise.

7. OPENING THE PALM

POSITION

Facing the hand.

Interlock one of your little fingers with the receiver's little finger and your thumb with his or her thumb. Bring your thumbs round onto the palm and make small circular movements all over the palm.

PURPOSE

■ Loosens the muscles and tendons.

■ Increases blood flow.

■ Eliminates accumulated waste products.

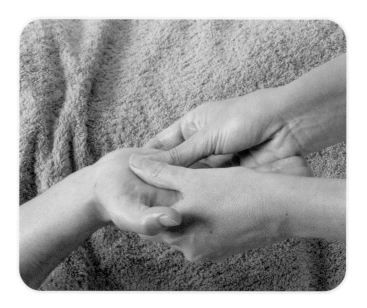

8. STROKING BETWEEN THE TENDONS

POSITION

Facing the hand.

Turn the hand over and hold the receiver's wrist to support the hand. Use the thumb of your free hand to work down the furrows between the tendons.

PURPOSE

■ Loosens the bones, tendons and muscle.

■ Breaks down adhesions and old scar tissue.

■ Releases toxins.

■ Increases blood flow to the hands.

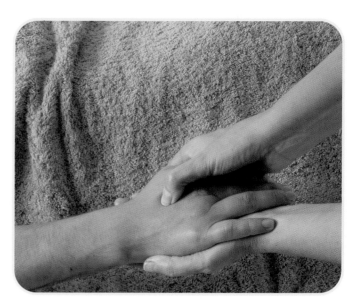

9. MASSAGING THE FINGERS

POSITION
Facing the hand.

PURPOSE
- Stimulates the blood supply to the fingers.
- Eliminates toxins.
- Prepares the fingers for mobilisation.

Support the hand and encircle the thumb and then each of the fingers in turn between your thumb and fingers. Gently stretch and perform a twisting corkscrew movement on each one.

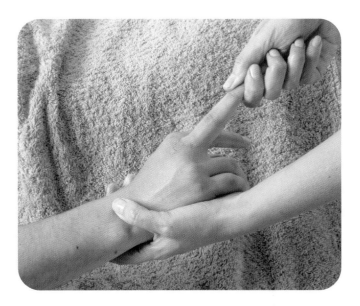

10. MOVING THE FINGERS

POSITION
Facing the hand.

PURPOSE
- Improves mobility of the finger joints.

Support the hand, and gently and slowly rotate the fingers and thumb individually clockwise and then anti-clockwise.

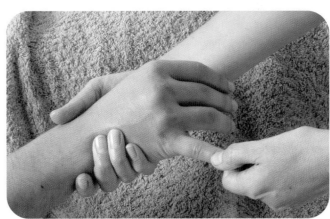

11. STROKING THE HAND AND ARM

POSITION
At the side of the receiver's arm.

PURPOSE
- Drains away toxins.
- Adds a finishing touch to the arm and hand massage.

Support the receiver's forearm underneath and effleurage up the arm with firm pressure several times. To finish the arm and hand massage, place your fingertips on the shoulder and perform fingertip stroking down the arm using just a feather-light touch.

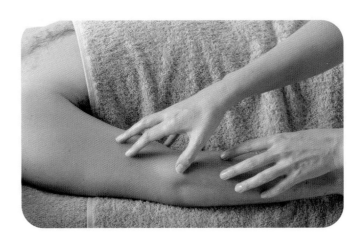

YOUR ARM AND HAND MASSAGE IS NOW COMPLETE

THE ABDOMEN

Uncover the abdomen in preparation for the massage. Tuck the top of the bottom towel into the receiver's underwear. Stand on the right hand side of the receiver to enable you to work around the colon in the correct direction. Tell the receiver not to talk or laugh since this tightens up the muscles and makes treatment difficult.

1. OILING

POSITION
On the right hand side of the receiver facing the abdomen.

PURPOSE
- Establishes the initial contact with the abdomen.
- Enables you to spread the massage oil.

Lower your hands gently down onto the abdomen, one palm on top of the other, and pause for a few moments since some individuals are apprehensive about having their abdomen massaged. Begin to move your hands in large clockwise circles around the abdomen. Your movements should be gentle and sensitive.

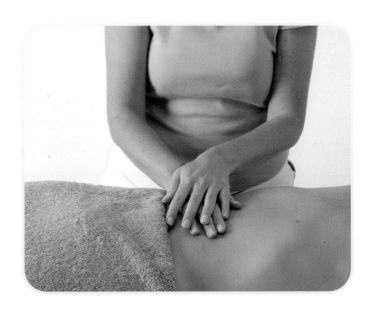

2. STROKING THE ABDOMEN

POSITION
On the right hand side of the receiver facing the abdomen.

PURPOSE
- Calms and soothes the abdomen.
- Helps to relieve digestive problems.
- Increases blood flow to the area.
- Assists detoxification.

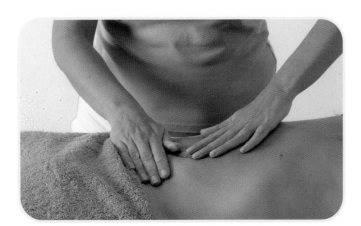

1. Place the palm of one hand on one side of the abdomen with the other on the opposite side. Effleurage around the abdomen in a clockwise direction, one hand following the other.

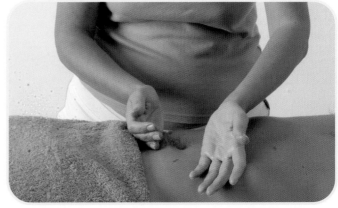

2. As a variation, try performing this movement using the back of your hand to perform the circular effleurage.

3. COLON FRICTIONING

POSITION

On the right hand side of the receiver, facing the abdomen.

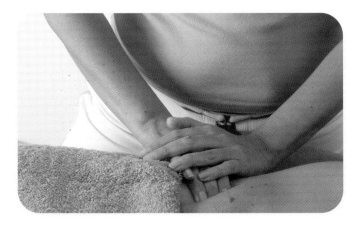

PURPOSE

- Relieves constipation.
- Stimulates the digestion.

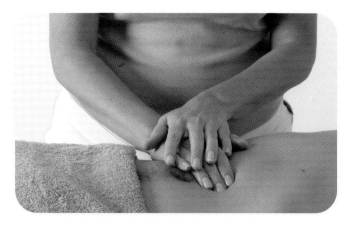

1. Place one hand palm downwards on the bottom right hand side of the abdomen and place the other hand gently on top. Using the pads of your fingers, perform small circular movements, working up the right-hand side of the abdomen. Make sure that you are not prodding it.

2. Continue your small pressure circles across the abdomen and then work down the left-hand side of the abdomen. Each time you friction the entire colon perform some effleurage.

4. DRAINING

POSITION

Facing the abdomen.

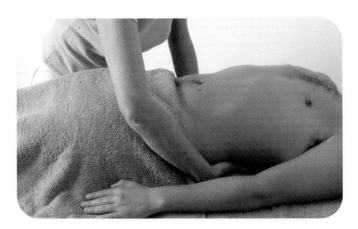

PURPOSE

- Reduces bloating.
- Drains toxins.

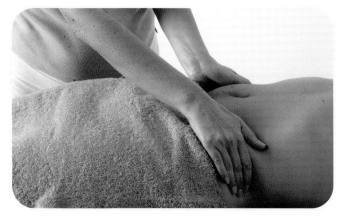

1. Place both hands, palms up, under the receiver's back, one from one side and one from the other side. Your fingertips may be touching.

2. Gently and slowly pull both hands up the sides of the abdomen and then diagonally down the abdomen.

5. KNEADING THE ABDOMEN

POSITION

Facing the abdomen.

PURPOSE

- Alleviates constipation.
- Improves the tone of the abdominal muscles.

Place one or both hands, palms downwards, flat on the abdominal area. Apply downward pressure (NOT a 'lifting' action as in the other petrissage movements) to perform kneading movements with the hands moving in the same or in opposite directions. The pressure is made alternately between the heel of the hand and the fingers.

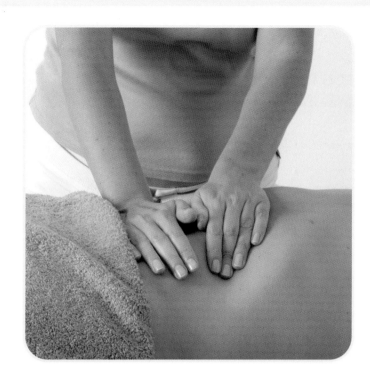

6. VIBRATING THE ABDOMEN

POSITION

Facing the abdomen.

PURPOSE

- Improves tone.
- Relieves flatulence, indigestion and constipation.
- Reduces pain.

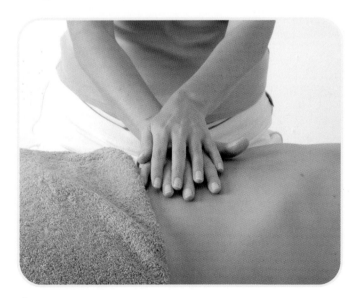

1. Place your hands, one on top of the other on the abdomen and then vibrate your hands rapidly yet gently from side to side.

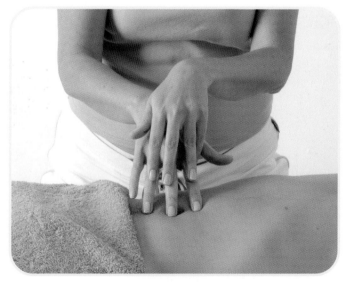

2. Now try the same movement using your fingertips rather than the whole of your hand. Place the fingertips of both hands below the navel and perform gentle vibrations taking care not to prod into the abdomen.

7. FINGERTIP STROKING

POSITION

On the right hand side of the receiver facing the abdomen.

PURPOSE

- Soothes and relaxes.
- Creates the final touch.

Use just your fingertips to stroke around the abdomen in a clockwise direction with one hand following the other. Let your movements become softer and softer until you are no longer touching the body.

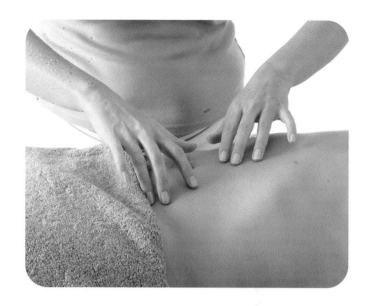

YOUR ABDOMINAL MASSAGE IS NOW COMPLETE

THE FRONT OF THE LEG AND FOOT

1. OILING

POSITION

At the side of the leg to be massaged.

PURPOSE

- Establishes contact with the leg.
- Spreads the massage oil.

Draw back the towel exposing only the leg to be treated. Dispense a small amount of warmed oil onto one hand and rub your palms together. Place both hands, palms downwards, gently onto the receiver's leg and stroke the oil onto the leg making sure that it is evenly spread.

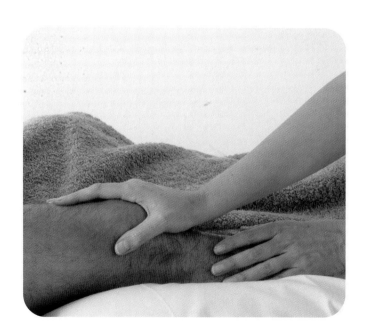

2. STROKING THE LEG

POSITION
At the side of the leg to be massaged.

PURPOSE
■ Stimulates circulation.

■ Eliminates toxins.

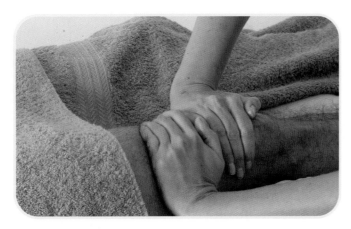

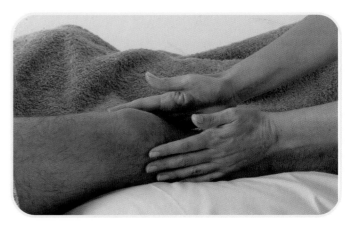

1. Place one hand across the receiver's ankle with the fingertips pointing in one direction and your other hand just above, with your fingertips pointing in the other direction. Effleurage slowly up the leg going lightly over the knee yet using a firm pressure on the thigh.

2. As you reach the top of the leg allow your hands to divide and glide them back to their starting position using no pressure. Repeat this movement several times.

3. DRAINING THE LOWER LEG

POSITION
At the receiver's foot.

PURPOSE
■ Drains the front of the leg.

■ Loosens the muscles.

■ Brings fresh blood to the area.

Make a 'V'-shape between your fingers and thumbs and place your hands just over the front of the ankle. Stroke up the leg from the ankle to just below the knee and then use alternate hands to perform the stroking movements. As one hand reaches the knee, lift it off and allow your other hand to take over the movement.

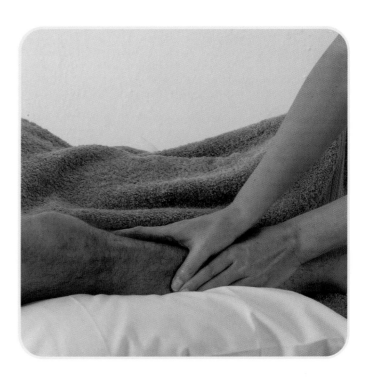

4. CIRCLING AND LOOSENING THE KNEECAP (PATELLA)

PURPOSE

- Loosens the knee joint.
- Releases and eliminates toxins.
- Breaks down old scar tissue.

POSITION

At the side of the knee.

1. Place the crossed tips of both thumbs just below the kneecap. Use the tip of your left thumb to circle anti-clockwise around the entire kneecap. Repeat several times and then use your right thumb to circle in a clockwise direction around the patella.

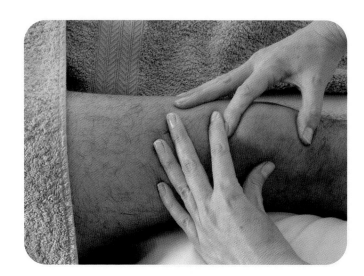

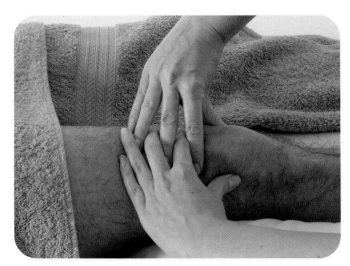

2. Now move both thumbs at the same time in exactly the same way as you did when you moved them separately. Repeat these circles about seven times.

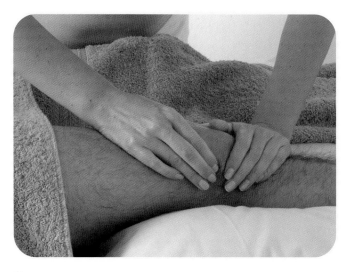

3. To loosen the patella further, use the pads of your thumbs to make small circular movements all around the knee joint.

5. DRAINING THE THIGH

POSITION
At the side of the thigh.

PURPOSE
- Drains away toxins.
- Prepares the thigh for deeper movements.
- Increases blood flow to the area.

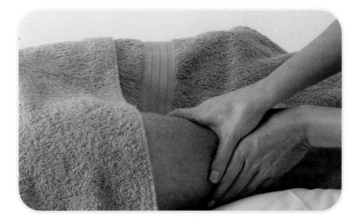

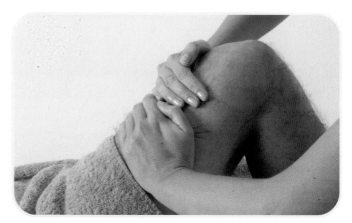

1. Make a 'V'-shape and place both hands, palms downwards, just above the knee. Use alternate hands to effleurage from the knee to the top of the leg making sure that you cover all aspects of the thigh.

2. As a variation, bend the knee and rest the foot on the massage surface. Place both hands just above the knee and stroke firmly up towards the thigh. This technique may be performed working both hands together or with alternate hands.

6. WRINGING THE THIGH

POSITION
At the side of the thigh.

PURPOSE
- Eliminates toxins.
- Breaks down fatty deposits.
- Improves circulation.
- Relieves muscular tension.

Use alternate hands to pick up and wring the muscles of the inner, middle and outer thigh. Work more gently on the sensitive inner thigh area, and deeply and strongly on the muscles of the outer thigh.

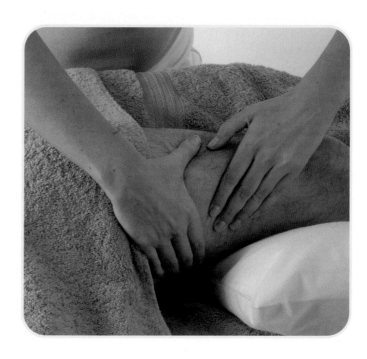

7. PERCUSSION OF THE THIGH

POSITION

At the side of the thigh.

PURPOSE

- Improves muscle tone in the thighs.
- Reduces fatty deposits and cellulite.
- Stimulates the circulation.
- Enlivens the whole body.

Women particularly adore percussion of the thigh as it reduces unsightly lumps and bumps. Percussion movements should not be performed on the lower leg since it is too bony and ensitive.

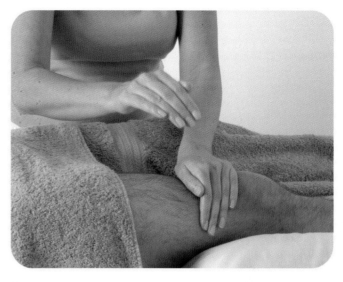

1. Form a hollow curve with both hands and hold them, palms facing downwards, just above the thigh. Bring your cupped hands down onto the thigh in quick succession. Keep your movements light and bouncy. Listen for a hollow sound – if you hear a slapping noise you need to cup your hands more.

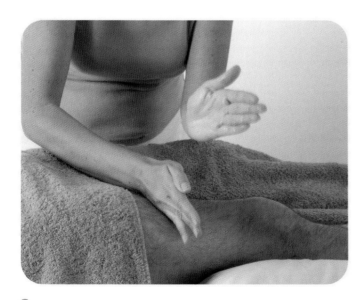

2. Shake your hands out to loosen the wrists and hold your hands over the thigh with the palms facing each other, thumbs uppermost. Flick them rapidly up and down onto the thigh in quick succession using the sides of your hands. Keep your movements bouncy, light and rhythmical.

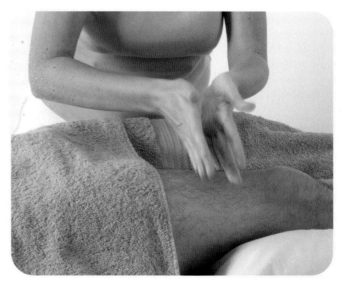

3. Place your hands, palms facing each other, thumbs uppermost over the thigh. Using the edge of the little fingers only, let your hands come down on the upper back in a series of rapid light strikes. This produces a much softer effect than the hacking.

>>

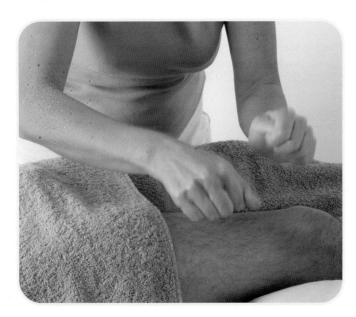

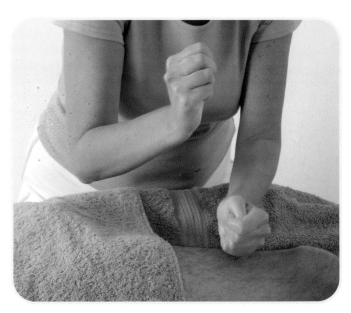

4. Make your hands into loose fists and, with hands and wrists relaxed, bring the palmar aspects of the fist in contact with the thigh to produce pounding.

5. Still with your fists loosely clenched, bounce the sides of your fists alternately against the thigh. This is beating.

8. FINGERTIP STROKING

POSITION

At the foot of the receiver.

PURPOSE

■ Induces a deep sense of relaxation.

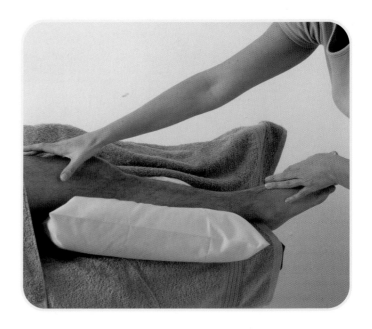

Place the fingertips of one hand at the top of the thigh and stroke gently down with a feather-light touch. As one hand reaches the foot lift it off gently whilst commencing the fingertip stroking with the other hand. To the receiver, it should feel like one continuous stroke. Stroke more and more gently continuing for as long as you like.

9. STROKING THE FOOT

According to reflexology, the foot is a mini map of the entire body. Therefore, as we massage the feet we are affecting all the rest of the body. The movements for the foot are very similar to the hand, so you should find this sequence fairly easy to master.

POSITION

Facing the receiver's foot.

PURPOSE

■ Establishes contact with the foot.

■ Assists the circulation.

■ Eliminates toxins.

■ Prepares the foot for deeper movements.

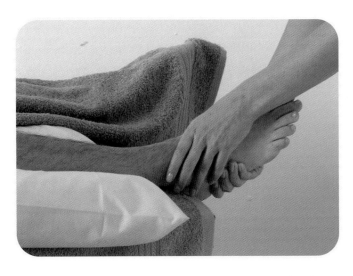

Use just a tiny amount of oil to stroke the foot. Sandwich the foot between your hands, fingers pointing upwards, and stroke firmly up the foot, gliding back gently with no pressure.

10. OPENING OUT THE SOLE OF THE FOOT

POSITION

Opposite the foot.

PURPOSE

■ Loosens muscles and tendons.

■ Breaks down adhesions.

■ Stimulates circulation to the entire body.

■ Eliminates waste products.

Wrap one hand around the top of the foot, make a loose fist with the other and place it on the fleshy area of the ball of the foot. Perform slow circular movements all over the sole.

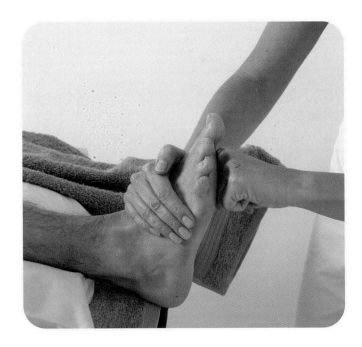

11. LOOSENING THE TOP OF THE FOOT

POSITION

Opposite the foot.

PURPOSE

- Loosens the muscles and tendons on top of the foot.
- Breaks down adhesions.
- Increases blood flow.
- Releases toxins.

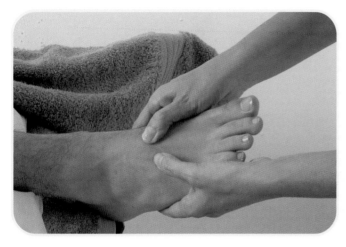

1. Place your fingers underneath the foot and each thumb on top just above the toes.

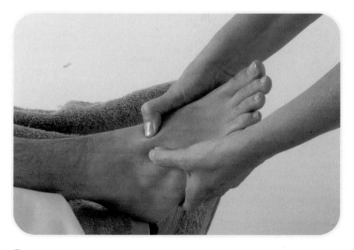

2. Perform firm, outward, circular movements using alternate thumbs and working up towards the ankle.

13. LOOSENING AND MOVING THE ANKLE

POSITION

Opposite the foot.

PURPOSE

- Improves mobility in the ankle.
- Breaks down knots and nodules.

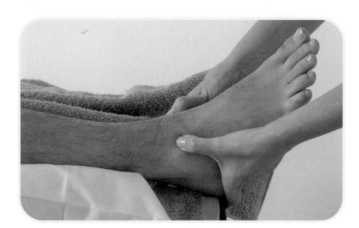

1. Use both thumbs, either alternately or together, to perform deep circular movements all around the ankle. Pay extra attention to areas that feel tight by frictioning deeply over them.

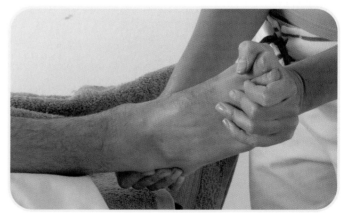

2. Support the foot underneath with one hand and use your other hand to circle the ankle both clockwise and anti-clockwise.

13. LOOSENING AND MOVING THE TOES

POSITION

Opposite the foot.

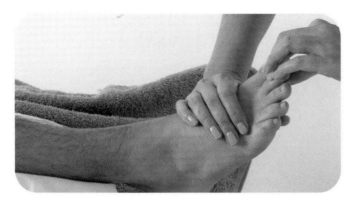

1. Support the foot by placing your thumb on the sole and fingers on top of the foot. Use the thumb and index finger of the other hand to massage each toe individually.

PURPOSE

- Encourages flexibility of the toes.
- Improves blood flow.
- Eliminates toxins.

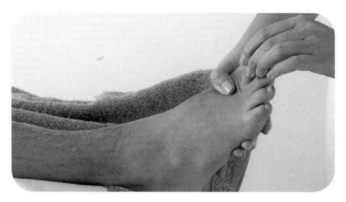

2. With your thumb and index finger circle each toe individually clockwise and then anti-clockwise.

THE FINAL TOUCH

Clasp the foot gently between your hands, one hand on the sole and one on the top. Hold this position for a few moments and then glide your hands very gently and slowly off the end of the toes.

After you have taken your hands away from the body try not to disturb the receiver for a few minutes. Cover him or her with an extra towel, move quietly and give them the opportunity to remain in this deeply relaxed state for as long as they like.

Always offer your massage partner a glass of water and advise him or her to drink plenty of water to assist the detoxification process.

POSITION

Opposite the foot.

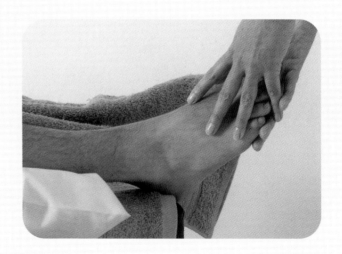

YOU HAVE NOW COMPLETED A FULL-BODY MASSAGE.

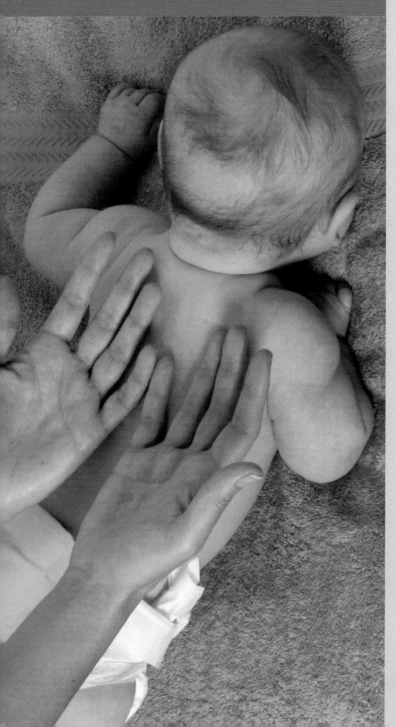

CHAPTER 4

MASSAGE FOR DIFFERENT OCCASIONS

MASSAGE FOR DIFFERENT OCCASIONS

MASSAGE FOR BABIES

EVERYONE CAN BENEFIT FROM THE HEALING POWER OF THE ANCIENT ART OF MASSAGE, EVEN THE VERY YOUNG. THERE IS NO BETTER START IN LIFE THAN THE WARMTH AND SECURITY THAT A BABY MASSAGE PROVIDES.

Babies who are massaged are generally much more contented, less fractious, suffer less colic and sleep much better. Their immune systems are also much stronger and a wonderful bond between parents and child is firmly established.

The following sequence is for a quick and simple baby massage. There are no special techniques; it is just a matter of adapting the strokes you have learnt and your hands for a tiny baby. It can be performed at any time of the day provided baby is in the right mood! A popular time is after bathing or after a night time feed.

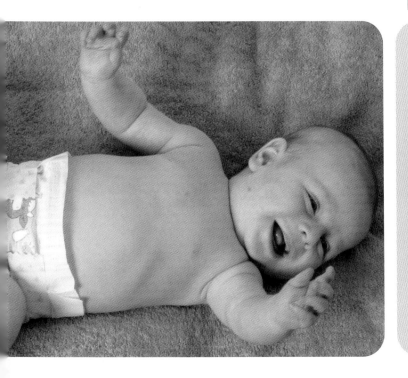

PREPARATION

- Warm the room as babies feel the cold more quickly than adults.
- Keep a spare blanket on hand to cover up baby.
- Keep a spare towel to clear up any little accidents!
- Check your nails are short and clean.
- Remove jewellery.
- Warm your hands.
- Prepare your oil. Remember, baby oil is a mineral oil and is not suitable for massage. Sweet almond oil is a popular choice. You can even make up an aromatherapy blend – try one drop of lavender and one drop of chamomile diluted in 15 ml (3 teaspoons) of carrier oil.
- Place a padded surface such as a changing mat or duvet on the floor and cover it with a soft warm towel.

SEQUENCE

Each movement should be repeated several times.

FACE

The face is an excellent place to begin your massage as you can have eye contact with your baby as they become accustomed to your strokes. Baby should lie on his or her back while you massage the front of the body.

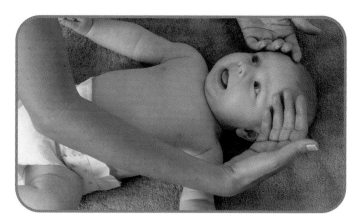

1. Use your fingertips to stroke baby's forehead from the centre outwards.

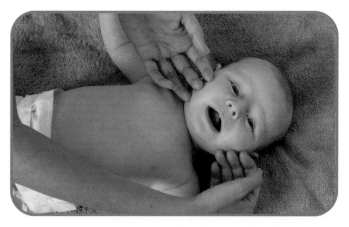

2. Then stroke from the nose outwards across the cheeks.

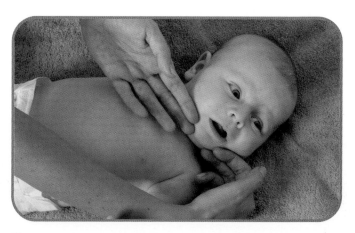

3. Now place your fingertips under the lips and stroke outwards across the chin.

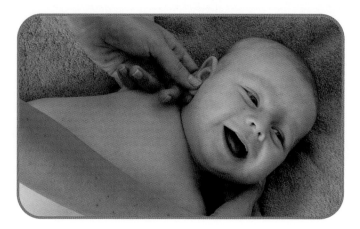

4. Massage and squeeze the ears very gently.

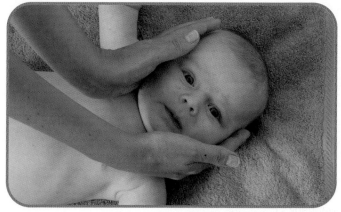

5. To complete baby's face massage, use feather-like strokes with your fingertips across the forehead and down the sides of the face.

CHEST

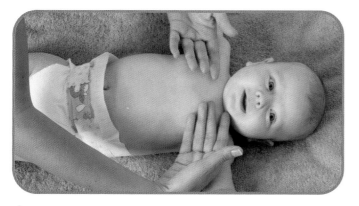

1. Place your hands in the centre of baby's upper chest, palms facing upwards, and stroke gently outwards towards the arms.

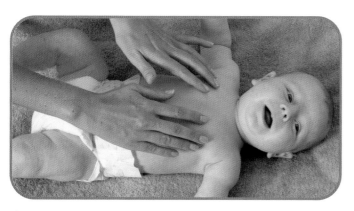

2. Use flat fingers to circle all over the chest.

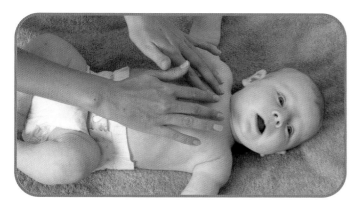

3. With the pads of your fingertips, tap very, very lightly all over baby's chest. This is excellent for loosening mucus and building up baby's immune system.

ABDOMEN

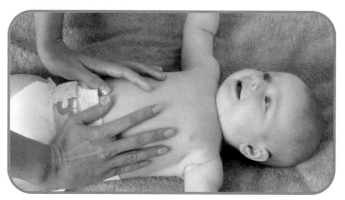

1. Rest both hands on baby's abdomen, one on either side of the navel.

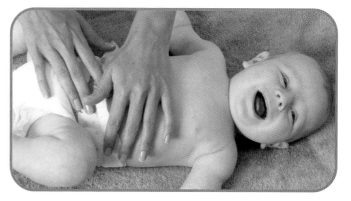

2. Circle slowly around the navel in a clockwise direction. As the hands cross over, lift one hand over the other. This movement is useful for relieving colic and digestive upsets.

ARMS

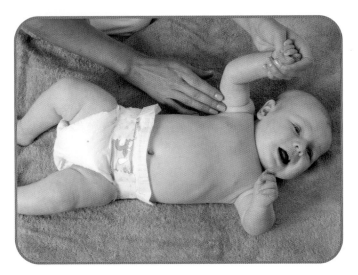

1. Hold baby's hand and stroke down the arm from the fingers to the shoulder.

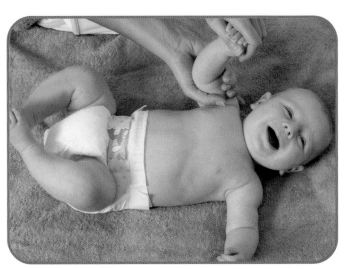

2. Wrap your fingers and thumb around baby's wrist and very gently squeeze and release all the way up to the shoulder.

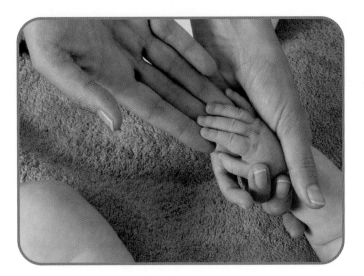

3. Support baby's hand at the wrist and use fingertip stroking on the back and the front of the hand.

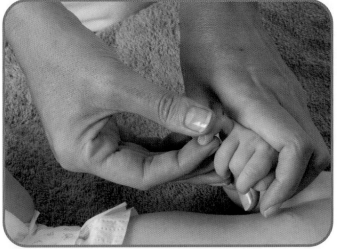

4. Gently massage baby's fingers and thumb by unfolding each one individually and circle each one in both directions. Repeat this sequence on the other arm.

LEGS

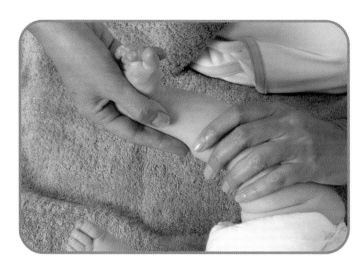

1. Lift baby's leg and hold the foot in one hand and stroke up the leg from foot to thigh. Allow your hands to glide back with no pressure.

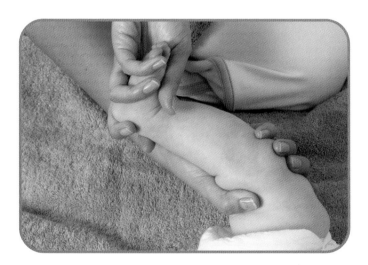

2. Wrap your fingers and thumb lightly around baby's ankle and squeeze and release from the foot to the top of the thigh.

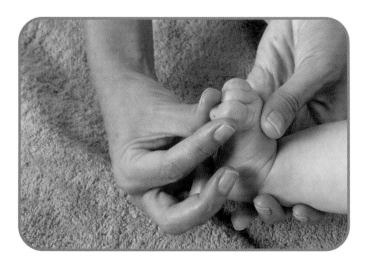

3. Gently squeeze each toe between your thumb and index finger and circle each one individually. Repeat this sequence on the other leg.

BACK

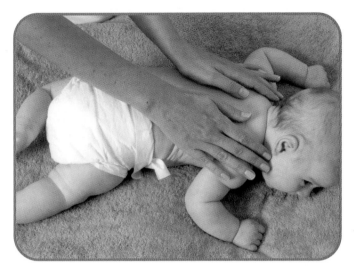

1. Turn baby over onto his or her tummy. Oil your hands and place them on the bottom of baby's back. Stroke gently up the back, over the shoulders and then allow them to glide back with a feather-light touch.

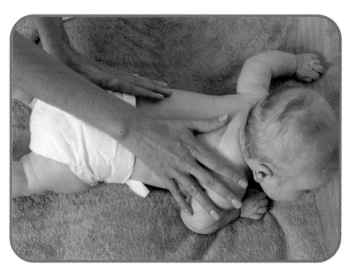

2. Once again, place both hands at the bottom of the back, one either side of the spine. Stroke one hand up the back and over the shoulder. Then lift it off gently and begin stroking with the other hand.

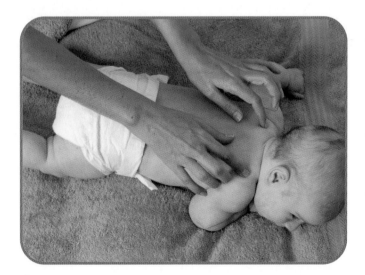

3. Place the pads of your fingertips at the top of baby's back either side of the spine. Tap very lightly down the back and then up again.

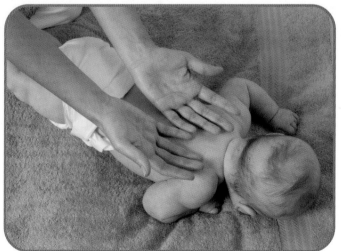

4. Complete the baby massage by gliding the backs of your hands from the head, down the back and over the legs.

MASSAGE FOR PREGNANCY

MASSAGE IS A SAFE AND NATURAL WAY TO PROMOTE A HEALTHY PREGNANCY AND TO ALLEVIATE ANY MINOR DISCOMFORTS WITHOUT THE USE OF DRUGS, WHICH ARE OFTEN CONTRAINDICATED AT THE TIME DUE TO THE RISK OF SIDE EFFECTS.

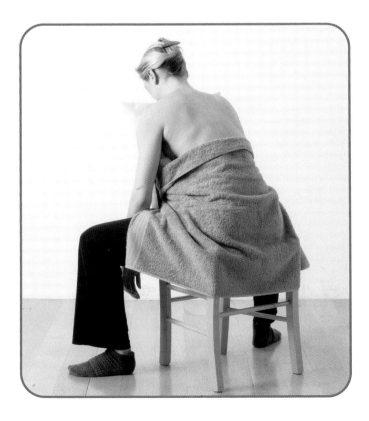

In the early stages of pregnancy, symptoms such as morning sickness, tiredness, headaches and mood swings are common. In later pregnancy, backache, fluid retention, varicose veins, cramps and indigestion are some of the problems that may be experienced. Massage can help to alleviate all of these problems. In my opinion massage is essential during pregnancy and in many years of practice I have always massaged and managed to prevent the dreaded stretch marks!

The following precautions should be observed:
- Only use gentle pressure – lots of effleurage and no percussion movements.
- Take extra special care over the abdomen and low back area.
- If there is a history of miscarriage massage should only be given with medical consent in the first three months.
- Complications such as high blood pressure, anaemia, diabetes and any vaginal bleeding should always be referred to a medical practitioner.

In the initial stages it is possible to carry out the step-by-step massage sequence already described. You will need to omit the tapotement and remember to use gentle pressure over the abdomen and low back. However, in later pregnancy, it will not be comfortable to lie on the stomach. One of the following positions is recommended:

1. Receiver sits astride a chair using cushions to fully support the abdomen. This is an ideal position for back, shoulder and neck massage.

2. Receiver lies on one side with her upper knee bent and resting on a pillow. Her head should also rest on a pillow.

3. Receiver lies on her back with pillows/cushions under the knees to relax the abdomen and reduce the curve in the lower back. Pillows should also be placed under the head. Use this position for massaging any area on the front of the body.

SEQUENCE

BACK

A back massage, in the later stages of pregnancy is best performed most easily in the sitting position. However, if the pregnant woman wants to lie down, then the side-lying position should be adopted. Both positions are just as beneficial, although the seated position is best for your back! The following sequence is carried out with the receiver seated.

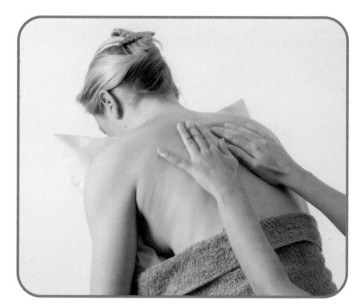

1. Kneel or stand behind the receiver and place both hands on the back, fingers pointing upwards. Stroke up the back around the shoulders and glide back to your starting position with no pressure whatsoever.

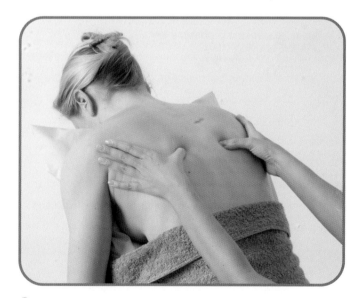

2. Place the pads of your thumbs on the receiver's back, one either side of the spine, and perform gentle circular movements working all the way up to the neck. This will help to break down any knots and nodules.

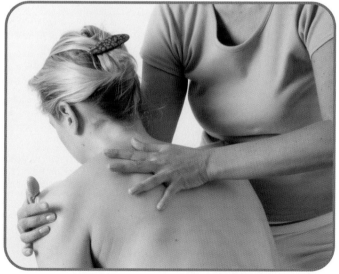

3. Stand at the side of the receiver. To work on the left shoulder blade place your right hand across the front of the body on top of the left shoulder and the palm of your left hand on the left shoulder blade. Circle around the shoulder with the palmar surface of your hand several times to warm and loosen it.

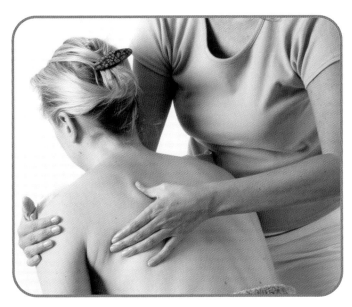

4. Keep the same position, but place the thumb of your left hand at the bottom of the left shoulder blade. Perform small, deep, circular movements all around the scapula to break down any knots and nodules.

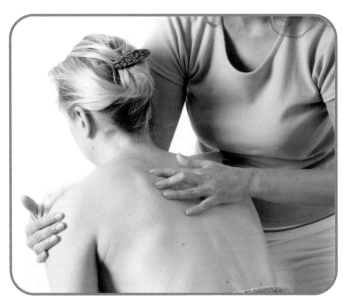

5. For a more gentle friction use your fingers instead of your thumb. Repeat steps 3 and 4 around the other shoulder blade.

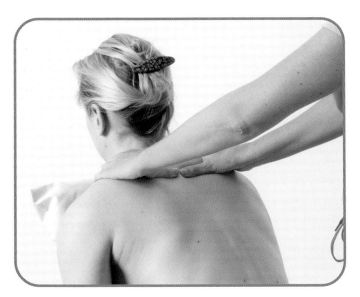

6. Stand behind the receiver and place the palms of both hands on the shoulder. Use alternate hands to rhythmically squeeze, pick up and wring the shoulder muscles.

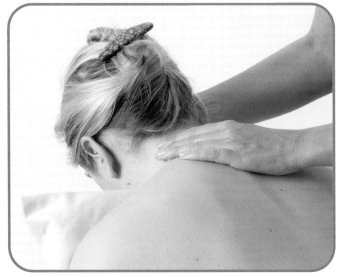

7. Stand to one side of the receiver. Place one hand on the forehead for support and place the other hand, palm downwards, on the back of the neck. Pick up and squeeze the muscles of the neck gently and slowly to release tension.

ABDOMEN

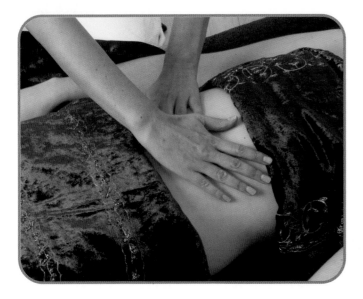

POSITION

The pregnant woman should lie on her back well supported by cushions and pillows.

PURPOSE

Abdominal massage is excellent for preventing stretch marks and for relieving taut skin. It is marvellous for constipation, eases sickness and heartburn and is ideal to encourage the bonding of mother and baby. Remember that pressure should be very gentle.

TECHNIQUE

Place both hands gently down onto the abdomen and stroke around the abdomen in a clockwise direction with one hand on top of the other. Place your hands, one either side of the abdomen, and stroke in a clockwise direction with one hand following the other. Place your hands, palms up, under the receiver's back, one under each side. Stroke very gently up the sides of the abdomen. To complete your abdominal massage use your fingertips to stroke softly in a clockwise direction around the abdomen, barely touching the skin.

LEGS AND FEET

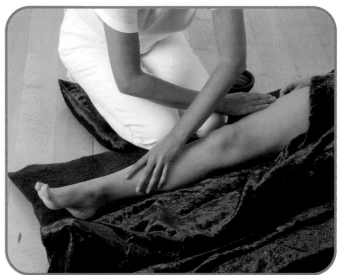

POSITION

The legs and feet can be massaged with the mother-to-be lying on her back with cushions under her knees and head.

PURPOSE

Leg massage is wonderful for preventing varicose veins and cramp, relieving fluid retention assisting the circulation and is also deeply relaxing.

TECHNIQUE

You can follow the sequence for the leg and foot as described on pages 69–75 and 97–105. For a simple treatment, place one hand on each ankle and stroke the legs gently from the ankles to the thighs. Glide the hands back with a feather-light touch.

ARMS AND HANDS

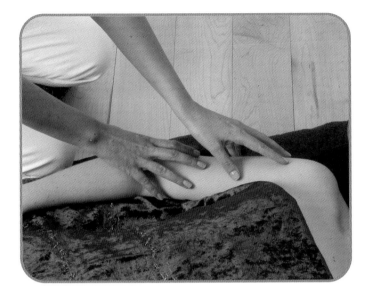

FACE

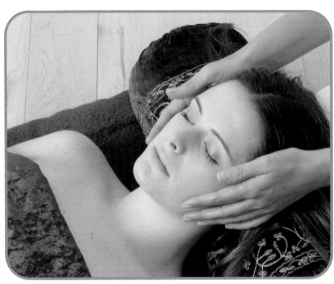

TECHNIQUE

You can massage the arms and hands as described on pages 89–93. Alternatively, you can simply effleurage the arms.

TECHNIQUE

Face massage is wonderfully relaxing and soothing. Follow the sequence on pages 84–88.

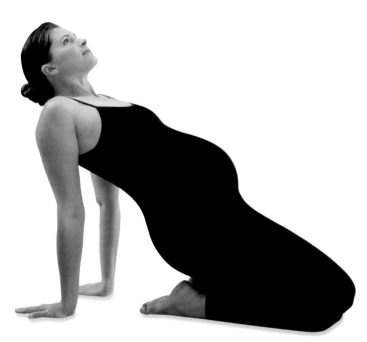

Massage is also highly beneficial for new mothers after they have given birth. In many cultures women are massaged daily after the birth. It helps to speed up recovery from the demands of pregnancy and childbirth. Massage helps the body to get back into shape both internally as well as externally. It promotes energy and vitality and prevents postnatal depression.

Follow the complete step-by-step sequence as described in this book. However, do not massage the scar area after a caesarean section and, even after a normal delivery, use only gentle stroking on the abdomen.

MASSAGE IN THE WORKPLACE

MASSAGE IS BECOMING INCREASINGLY POPULAR IN THE WORKPLACE. A SHORT 10–15 MINUTES OF MASSAGE CAN BE REMARKABLY INVIGORATING AND IS THE PERFECT WAY TO DE-STRESS AND IMPROVE YOUR POWERS OF CONCENTRATION.

To save time the massage can be performed through clothes. All you need is a chair that enables you to reach the head and shoulders comfortably without having to bend or strain, and a willing partner!

Try out this simple 10-minute sequence on your colleagues.

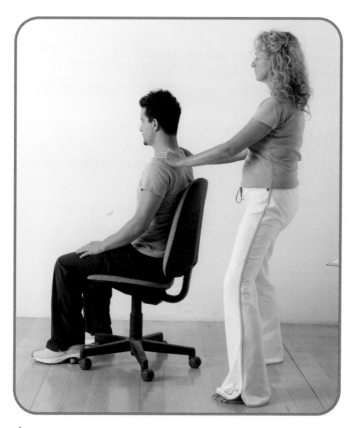

1. Ask your partner to sit comfortably in a chair, legs uncrossed and feet flat on the ground. Stand squarely behind them place your hands on top of their shoulders and ask them to take a few deep breaths. Ask them to breathe in energy and vitality and to breathe out tiredness and tension.

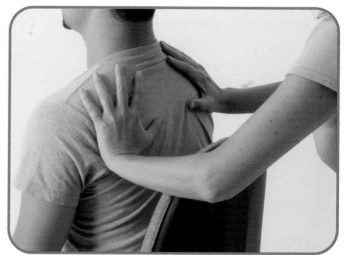

2. Place a hand on each shoulder blade and perform large, stroking,circular movements over both scapulae. This will loosen tight muscles and warm up the back and shoulders.

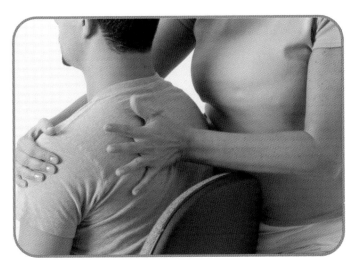

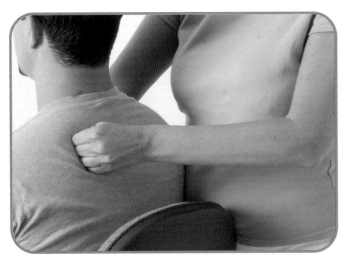

3. Position yourself at the receiver's right side. Place your right arm over the front of the receiver's left shoulder and place the whole of your left hand on the left scapula. Rub lightly and briskly all over the shoulder blade area to bring fresh blood and nutrients to the area, boost the lymphatic circulation and to loosen tight muscles.

4. In the same position as for step 3 make a loose fist and use your knuckles to work all around the shoulder blade paying particular attention to any knots and nodules. Repeat steps 3 and 4 on the other shoulder blade.

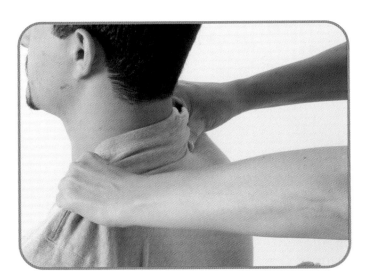

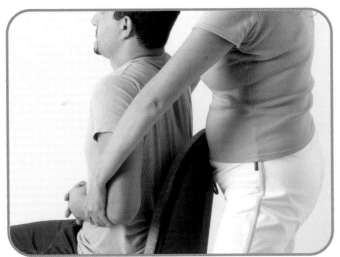

5. Place one hand on the top of each shoulder and squeeze and release the shoulder muscles to relieve stiffness and tightness.

6. Stand behind the receiver and ask him or her to rest their hands in their lap. Place your hands under their elbows and then lift their arms and shoulders. Hold for a few seconds and then release them.

>>

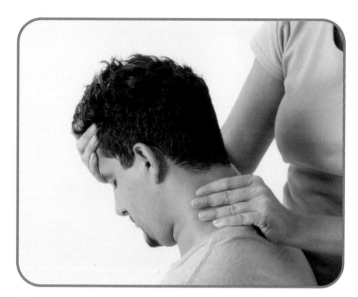

7. Stand to the side of the receiver. Let his or her forehead drop into one hand and place your other hand on the back of the neck in a V-shape. Squeeze the neck muscles between your thumb and fingers to melt away stress and anxiety.

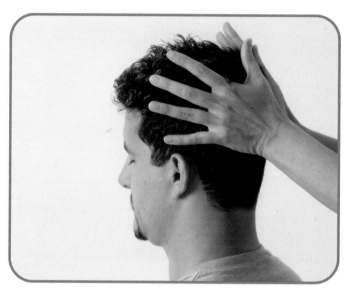

8. Positioned squarely behind the receiver, place your hands on either side of the head. Use the heels of your hands to circle over the sides, top and back of the scalp to release tension.

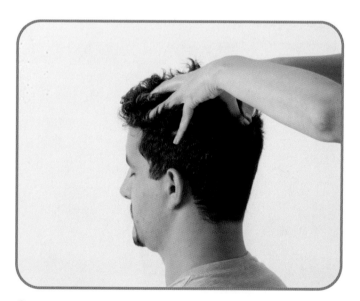

9. Make claw-like shapes with your hands and place them on the top of the head. Use the pads of your fingers and thumbs to perform small, slow, circular movements all over the scalp. Your pressure should be fairly firm and, as you work, you should begin to feel the scalp move as the tension dissipates.

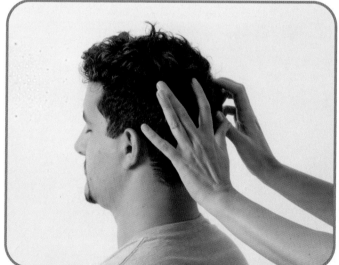

10. Hold your hands just above the receiver's scalp and tap the pads of your fingers all over the receiver's scalp and the back of the neck. Make your movements quick, bouncy and energetic to revitalise and awaken your colleague. They should now feel relaxed and refreshed and ready to continue with the day.

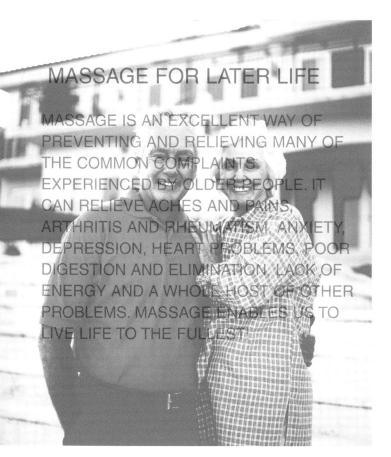

MASSAGE FOR LATER LIFE

MASSAGE IS AN EXCELLENT WAY OF PREVENTING AND RELIEVING MANY OF THE COMMON COMPLAINTS EXPERIENCED BY OLDER PEOPLE. IT CAN RELIEVE ACHES AND PAINS, ARTHRITIS AND RHEUMATISM, ANXIETY, DEPRESSION, HEART PROBLEMS, POOR DIGESTION AND ELIMINATION, LACK OF ENERGY AND A WHOLE HOST OF OTHER PROBLEMS. MASSAGE ENABLES US TO LIVE LIFE TO THE FULLEST.

When working on older people it is vital that the room is warm since many of them feel the cold very easily. They may even wish to keep their clothes on. Try to be sensitive to the needs of the individual.

The areas which are most accessible are the hands and feet. Older people derive great benefit from having these areas massaged. Arthritis is usually a problem and pain can be considerably relieved by the use of massage. A treatment of the hands or feet is an excellent introduction to massage for the elderly. The neck, shoulders, back and knees are also areas that are prone to stiffness and respond well to treatment.

Older people will find treatment on a massage couch quite acceptable, but may find it uncomfortable to lie on the floor. Therefore, if you do not have a massage table it is probably best to carry out treatments with the receiver on a chair. You need to be very adaptable and be prepared to roll garments up and to sometimes work through the clothes. It's well worth the effort – the elderly adore massage.

DOS AND DON'TS

- Do check for contraindications.
- Do use gentle pressure as older skin tends to be thinner and more fragile.
- Do massage above and below swollen areas.
- Do massage unaffected joints to improve mobility.
- Do advise checking out any suspicious lumps or moles.
- Do use more massage oil as elderly skin tends to be dryer.
- Do check with the doctor as to the advisability of massage if there is a medical condition such as osteoporosis, cardiac disease etc.

- Do take care with diabetics. The peripheral circulation can be poor and, if the nerves are affected, there may be a loss of sensory function so that the elderly person will not be able to give you accurate feedback.
- Don't massage directly on inflamed joints.
- Don't perform any vigorous stretching.
- Don't mobilise painful joints.
- Don't massage severe varicose veins.

SIMPLE HAND MASSAGE SEQUENCE

ACCORDING TO HAND REFLEXOLOGY, ALL THE ORGANS, GLANDS AND STRUCTURES OF THE BODY RELATE TO SPECIFIC AREAS OF THE HANDS; THEY ARE A MIRROR OF THE BODY. IF YOU MASSAGE THE HANDS YOU ARE TREATING THE WHOLE PERSON.

This sequence is for the left hand.

Make sure the receiver is relaxed and sitting comfortably on a chair. Ask them to remove their shoes and place their feet flat on the ground with the legs uncrossed. Place a pillow or cushion on their laps so that they can rest their hand on it. You may want to place a towel over the pillow to avoid oil stains.

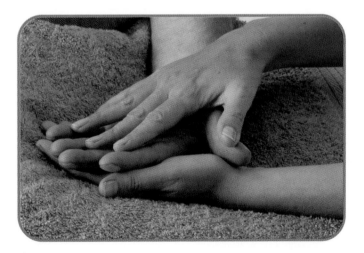

1. Take hold of the receiver's hand between both of yours. Clasp it very gently for a few moments. This will help to relax and reassure the person.

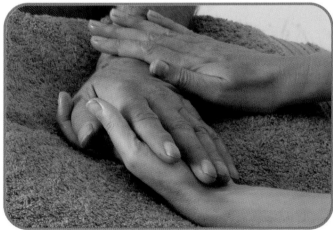

2. Support the wrist with your left hand and stroke up to the top of the hand. Repeat several times.

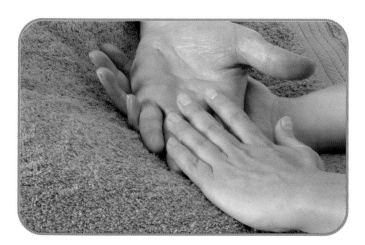

3. Then turn the hand over and stroke the palm. Gentle effleurage soothes, relaxes and improves the circulation.

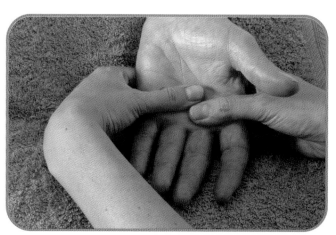

4. With their hand palm uppermost, place your fingers underneath the hand with thumbs parallel on top. Draw your thumbs out to the side gently opening up the palm of the hand. Repeat this movement on the entire palm and then turn the hand over and open up the back of the hand.

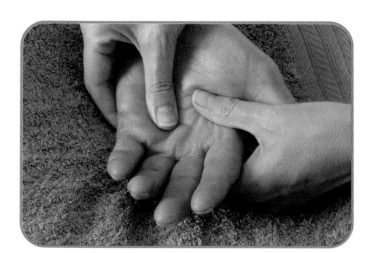

5. Supporting the wrist with your left hand, make small, round, circular movements all over the palm. This movement helps to loosen the muscles, tendons and joints. Make sure that you do not apply too much pressure.

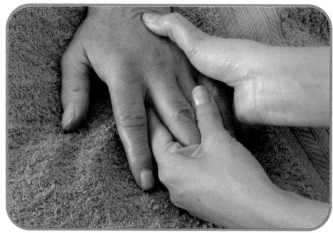

6. Turn the hand over and use the thumb, and index or middle finger to work along each of the furrows between the bones of the hands.

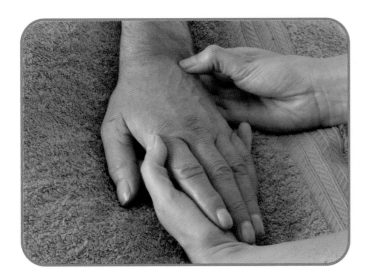

7. Support the hand and use the tips of your fingers to perform small, circular movements all around the wrist. Gentle friction helps to loosen up the wrist joint.

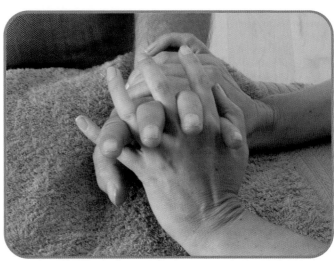

8. Support the wrist with one hand and interlock your fingers of the other hand with the receiver. Very gently and slowly move the wrist clockwise and then anti-clockwise. Do not try to force the wrist – it may not move very far.

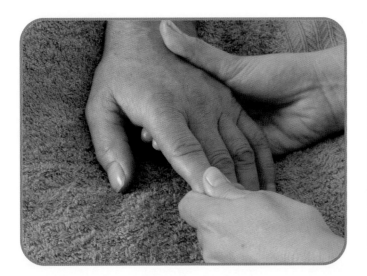

9. Hold the receiver's wrist with one hand and use the thumb and index finger of your other hand to gently and slowly stretch and squeeze the thumb and each of the fingers.

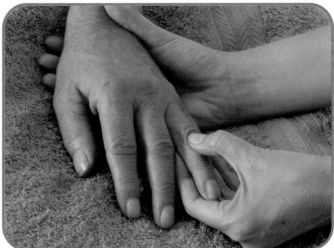

10. Support the wrist and, with your thumb on top and index finger underneath, circle very gently and slowly over each of the finger joints. This will increase mobility, relieve pain, eliminate toxins and increase the blood supply to the fingers.

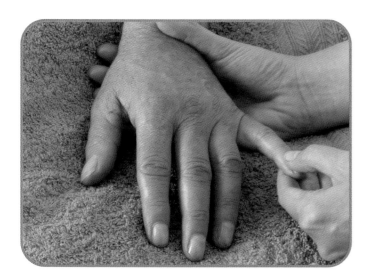

11. With your thumb and index finger, gently circle the thumb and fingers individually both clockwise and anti-clockwise. Remember not to force the joints.

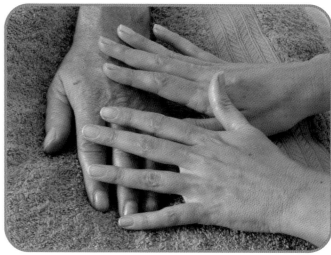

12. To complete the treatment, place the receiver's hand on the cushion and use your fingertips to stroke down the hand using barely any pressure. Repeat the entire sequence on the other hand. You will be amazed at the results!

It is highly beneficial for elderly people to massage their own hands every day as it will keep the skin thoroughly moisturised and soft and the hands wonderfully supple. Daily massage of the hands will also engender a sense of peace and well-being. Experiment with some of the essential oils mentioned in this book. Chamomile is highly recommended since it reduces inflammation, relieves aches and pains and calms and soothes.

Frankincense is also recommended as it revitalises and combats ageing skin. Geranium helps to boost the circulation and is very uplifting. Lemon assists with the removal of toxins and is an overall tonic. Rosemary is pain relieving and stimulates the mind.

The importance of a good diet for maintaining and preventing ill-health cannot be stressed enough. Fresh fruit and vegetables should be eaten daily and eight glasses of water are recommended. Gentle exercise, such as a short daily walk, is also essential. Regular moderate exercise will improve circulation, tone the muscles, keep the joints flexible and help to prevent many diseases such as osteoporosis and heart problems.

Try one of the following blends:

Dilute in 20 ml carrier oil two drops chamomile, two drops geranium and two drops lemon.

Dilute in 20 ml carrier oil three drops frankincense and three drops rosemary.

Three drops chamomile in a small bowl of warm water makes a soothing aromatherapy hand bath which will aid pain relief and lessen inflammation.

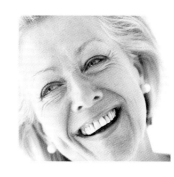

CONCLUSION

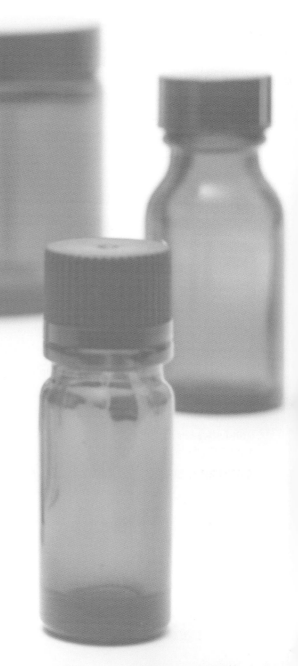

I do hope that you have enjoyed learning and practising the healing art of massage. Touch is truly magical and has enormous benefits for body, mind and spirit. Try to swap a massage regularly every week with a friend and you will notice a big difference in your health and well-being.

I may even have inspired some of you to train to be a professional massage therapist. Do make sure that you train with a reputable, long-established massage college that is accredited to a professional association. Visit the college to check out the standard of the work and talk to current students to discover if they are satisfied with the course. Massage therapy is a very rewarding occupation.

INDEX

USEFUL ADDRESSES

UK

BEAUMONT COLLEGE OF NATURAL MEDICINE

MWB Business Exchange
23 Hinton Road,
Bournemouth, BH1 2EF
Tel: +44 (0)1202 708887
www.beaumontcollege.co.uk
Information on professional training courses under the personal direction of Denise Whichello Brown.

DENISE BROWN ESSENTIAL OILS

Tel: +44 (0)1202 708887
www.denisebrown.co.uk
For a wide selection of high-quality, pure, unadulterated essential oils, base oils, creams and lotions, relaxation music, wall charts etc. (International Mail Order).

THE ASSOCIATION OF OSTEOMYOLOGISTS (MANUAL THERAPY)

80 Greenstead Avenue,
Woodford Green,
Essex IG8 7ER
Tel: +44 (0) 20 8504 1462
www.osteomyology.co.uk

THE SOCIETY OF HOMEOPATHS

4a Artizan Road, Northampton
NN1 4HU
Tel: +44 (0) 1604 621400
www.homeopathy-soh.org
The largest organisation registering professional homoeopaths in the UK.

BRITISH HOMEOPATHIC ASSOCIATION

15 Clerkenwell Close,
London EC1R 0AA
Tel: +44 (0) 20 7566 7800
www.trusthomeopathy.org
Helpful information about homeopathy.

OSTEOPATHIC CENTRE FOR CHILDREN

109 Harley Street,
London W1G 6AN
Tel: +44 (0) 20 7486 6160
www.occ.uk.com

INTEGRAL YOGA

293 Malmesbury Park Road
Charminster,
Bournemouth BH8 8PX
Tel: +44 (0) 1202 251548
Offers a wide range of classes.

WWW.HEALTHYPAGES.NET

A popular UK-based site, hosting information about courses, schools and therapists etc.

WWW.CHISUK.ORG.UK

Complementary Healthcare Information Service – UK based.

USA

WWW.ABOUTMASSAGE.COM

A site that has information on massage associations based in the USA.

AMERICAN ACADEMY OF OSTEOPATHY

www.academyofosteopathy.org
Telephone +1 (317) 879-1881-129

CREDITS

The author and publishers would like to thank the following models for their participation:
Caron Bosler
Alexis Henderson
Eduardo Henriquez
Felix Gilham (baby massage sequence)

Pictures pp 7–9, 13, 17, 117b © Getty Images
Pictures pp 125bl © Stockbyte
(where b=bottom, l=left)